Pranayama Lost in Translation

of related interest

Restoring Prana
A Therapeutic Guide to Pranayama and Healing Through the Breath
for Yoga Therapists, Yoga Teachers, and Healthcare Practitioners
Robin L. Rothenberg
Illustrated by Kirsteen Wright
Foreword by Richard Miller
ISBN 978 1 84819 401 4
eISBN 978 0 85701 357 6

Svadhyaya Breath Journal
A Companion Workbook to Restoring Prana
Robin L. Rothenberg
ISBN 978 1 78775 258 0

Yoga – Anticolonial Philosophy
An Action-Focused Guide to Practice
Shyam Ranganathan
ISBN 978 1 83997 876 0
eISBN 978 1 83997 877 7

Yoga Teaching Handbook
A Practical Guide for Yoga Teachers and Trainees
Edited by Sian O'Neill
ISBN 978 1 84819 355 0
eISBN 978 0 85701 313 2

PRANAYAMA
LOST IN TRANSLATION
From the Hatha Verses to Practice

Angela Andrea Ashwin

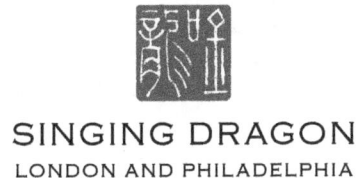

SINGING DRAGON
LONDON AND PHILADELPHIA

First published in Great Britain in 2025 by Singing Dragon,
an imprint of Jessica Kingsley Publishers
Part of John Murray Press

1

Copyright © Angela Andrea Ashwin 2025

The right of Angela Andrea Ashwin to be identified as the Author of the Work has been asserted by them in accordance with the Copyright, Designs and Patents Act 1988.

Illustrations © Melanie Hackett 2025
Front cover image source: iStockphoto®. The cover image is for illustrative purposes only, and any person featuring is a model.

All rights reserved. No part of this publication may be reproduced, stored in a retrieval system, or transmitted, in any form or by any means without the prior written permission of the publisher, nor be otherwise circulated in any form of binding or cover other than that in which it is published and without a similar condition being imposed on the subsequent purchaser.

The information contained in this book is not intended to replace the services of trained medical professionals or to be a substitute for medical advice. The complementary therapy described in this book may not be suitable for everyone to follow. You are advised to consult a doctor before embarking on any complementary therapy programme and on any matters relating to your health, and in particular on any matters that may require diagnosis or medical attention.

A CIP catalogue record for this title is available from the
British Library and the Library of Congress

ISBN 978 1 80501 734 9
eISBN 978 1 80501 735 6

Printed and bound in Great Britain by CPI Group

Jessica Kingsley Publishers' policy is to use papers that are natural, renewable and recyclable products and made from wood grown in sustainable forests. The logging and manufacturing processes are expected to conform to the environmental regulations of the country of origin.

Singing Dragon
Carmelite House
50 Victoria Embankment
London EC4Y 0DZ

www.singingdragon.com

John Murray Press
Part of Hodder & Stoughton Ltd
An Hachette Company

The authorised representative in the EEA is Hachette Ireland,
8 Castlecourt Centre, Dublin 15, D15 XTP3, Ireland (email: info@hbgi.ie)

Contents

Acknowledgements 9

Introduction 11
We seem to have forgotten what Yoga is and where it comes from 11
A different method: svadhyaya 15

1. Setting the Scene 19
   Yogis did not practise with their anatomical bodies 19
   Consciousness is not an anatomical process 21
   Life is not an anatomical process 22
   Pranayama is not an anatomical process 24
   Indian medical science did not work with the anatomical body 26
   Yoga works on deeper, non-physical dimensions 27

2. Hatha Yoga – the Tradition that Refined Pranayama 33
   The concept of Prana up to the Hatha times 33
   Prana is the 'Hatha Yoga anatomy' 35
   The historical journey of pranayama from Hatha to modern Yoga 39
   Lost in translation 41

3. Prana 43
   Samskaras determine the way a culture perceives the universe 44
   The great and the individual Prana, Maha Prana and vayu 45
   Prana and Atman 47
   Prana and breath 48

Nadi	49
Vayu (wind)	51
The five main vayus	52
The origin of vayu, manipura	58

4. Pranayama 69

How pranayama is often taught in modern Yoga	69
We have to be a scholar and a practitioner	76
Pranayama explained in the Hatha verses	78
Pranayama is the process of clearing the nadis	79
What are these impurities?	84
Common techniques used to facilitate pranayama	86
Agni sari	87
Ujjayi	88
Tadagi	89
Kabalabhati	89
Bastrika	91
Bhramari	92
Simbhasana	93
Viloma	95
Ratio breathing	95
Nadi sodhana	96
Does Hatha Yoga instruct pranayama techniques?	97
Verse 7	102
Verse 8	104
The eight kumbhakas	107
The link between Prana and citta	111
The goal of pranayama	112
What is kundalini?	114
Where is kundalini located?	116
Is Kundalini different from Prana?	117
What happens when kundalini awakens?	117
Do only special people have an awakened kundalini?	118

	How to awaken kundalini: the evidence in the Hatha compositions	119
	Pranayama in non-Hatha traditions	122
	Pranayama as described in Patanjali 2, 49-52	123
5.	**Bandhas**	129
	Mula bandha (MB)	132
	Uddiyana bandha (UB)	135
	Jalandhara bandha (JB)	137
6.	**Samadhi**	141
	Conclusion	145
	Glossary	147
	Bibliography	157

Acknowledgements

I never saw myself writing a book. I was convinced that I am a speaker, writing is not my thing. But I did write, I wrote many detailed handouts for my students on my Yoga teacher training courses in the absence of good course material. My first thank you goes therefore to those of you who valued my handouts and suggested I try to publish them. When I started to write with the intention of creating a book, I spoke to my uncle Werner Kelber, an author of many books himself as a professor for religious studies. He kindly read my first attempt and gave me the necessary confidence to continue. I very much thank Joy Simpson for proofreading the whole of this first attempt and giving me valuable feedback. This first attempt was a more general overview of the history of Yoga, and when I presented it to the theologian Ionut Moise he asked me which chapter I considered gave a new message and had a specific personal take. I said, 'the chapter on pranayama', and he advised me to make a whole book out of this chapter. This is what I did; Ionut, thanks for the advice. Special thanks go to my daughter Melanie Hackett, who took all the photographs for the book and drew the images. And finally thank you my dear friend Sharon Dow for proofreading the whole book during the editing process.

INTRODUCTION

We seem to have forgotten what Yoga is and where it comes from
Before the 1950s, few people in the Western world practised Yoga. When the discipline first came to the West, it was seen as mysterious, and we began to explain it using Western knowledge and scientific methods; in this way, it increasingly became a Westernized practice. In a sense, we stole Yoga from India and pretended it was ours.

Recently, I attended a coffee afternoon at a secondary school. I was talking to a 15-year-old boy, and he asked me what my profession was, so I told him that I am a Yoga teacher. He had heard of Yoga, and as we continued our conversation, I mentioned India, but the boy looked blank. He did not know that Yoga did not originate in the West. Perhaps, I thought, it is not so strange that a 15-year-old boy would be unaware of this. I relayed our conversation to one of the teachers, and to my astonishment, I found that the teacher was also unaware that Yoga has its origins in India – even though she had participated in Yoga classes. Upon realizing his misconception around the origins of Yoga, the boy remarked fittingly, 'That is twisted.' Today, Yoga is often taught as if it is a Western practice, using Western knowledge and science and with a Western worldview – we are twisting it into something it is not.

When I trained as a Yoga teacher, much of the teacher training course was spent on anatomy, analysing the muscles as they contracted or stretched in certain postures, and studying the respiratory system and the link between respiration, the heart and other body systems.

We discussed the physical benefits of all the Yoga practices in detail. Towards the end of the course, we looked at the so-called 'texts', the verses from the Indian Yoga tradition containing all the instructions and explanations of Yoga, verses that were composed thousands of years ago. The 'study of the texts' was the part of the syllabus called 'Yoga philosophy' and it was unrelated to the physical practice.

These verses are the explanations and instructions for the practice of Yoga. They have been passed down orally from Indian Yoga master to student from generation to generation. They express Yoga, instruct Yoga, show how Yoga developed throughout Indian history. The verses have always been an oral tradition. Today we have them in written form in Sanskrit and translated into our own languages. The verses we studied in the Yoga teacher training course were from the Upanishads, the Bhagavad Gita, the Patanjali Yoga Sutras and the Hatha Yoga Pradipika. These verses lay out the path of Yoga. I believe that these verses are our treasure; they are the tools to learn Yoga. They are not 'philosophy' unrelated to practice but are practical instructions.

What is 'philosophical' about the verses is that following their guidance leads to Self-realization, a deeply meaningful concept revealing the purpose of life. By practising the instructions in these verses, we realize that life is a journey, a path. We realize that we are here in this life, on this planet, to evolve and not just to keep this physical body going as long and as well as possible. This ancient Yoga tradition does not mention muscles and joints, respiration, lungs, oxygen intake or other body systems. The verses teach how to control the mind, how to reach enlightenment. They teach how to overcome the human obstacles of attachment and Ego, they speak about consciousness and the Divine, and they explain prana, chakras, nadis and kundalini. Instead of learning to teach mind control, enlightenment, overcoming the Ego, consciousness and the Divine, prana, nadis, chakras and kundalini in the Yoga teacher training course, we learned to teach muscular movements, techniques to enhance respiration and relaxation to undo stress responses. We received a physical therapy training unconnected to the so-called philosophy, which left three options:

1. To teach a physical practice focusing on human anatomy and discarding the philosophy. This path is probably taken by most Yoga teachers these days.
2. To continue to study the philosophy, attending courses, giving talks, writing articles or even books on the topic, becoming a scholar.

3. To try to understand that the 'practice' and the 'philosophy' are one and the same.

I have always tried to follow the third option. Like many Yoga teachers, I had the vague sense that asana is not just physical movement and pranayama is not just respiration. Throughout my teaching life, I have tried to integrate the old verses into my classes, which is a difficult undertaking. We are so heavily programmed in the Western way of viewing the body merely as a form composed of matter in need of repair that it seems incomprehensible that physical movement can lead to a spiritual opening. My attempt to connect the 'practice' and the 'philosophy' has been ongoing for the past 30 years, but the journey has become easier. Increasingly, the physical practice has become a way for me to work with our life force and the mind, working towards enlightenment, overcoming attachments and Ego, connecting to Consciousness and the Divine. I have learned to work with prana, nadis, chakras, kundalini and pranayama instead of muscles, nervous reactions and respiration.

As a Yoga teacher trainee assessor, I have travelled to student teachers' classes to give feedback on their teaching. I have seen many attempts to connect physical movement with spirituality. Some attempts were good; others were just physical classes with the reading of a quote at the beginning and the end of the class. Some attempts were moving; others were cheesy, using clichés devoid of personal experience.

The students in my teacher training courses are encouraged to enter the world of 'Indian thinking', to experience it in their own practice and to learn to pass the Indian message on to their students.

I was bewildered during my training by the disconnection of the Yoga teaching and the 'philosophy'. I was nevertheless lucky to study with the British Wheel of Yoga, who taught some of the so-called 'Yoga philosophy' – many Yoga teacher training courses today have excluded it from the syllabus. We were encouraged to add a 'theme' into each class; this usually meant reading a verse from the Yoga tradition, which was followed by posture work with occasional reference to the meaning of the verse, followed by breathing practice and a relaxation. We all loved the meaningful verses but did not really understand how they related to the 'Yoga' we learned to teach. Those meaningful verses *are* Yoga!

It seemed to be so difficult to teach Yoga and relate it to the Indian tradition. In other words, it seemed so difficult to teach Yoga and relate it to Yoga.

To discover Yoga, we need to 'unlearn' our Western programming which perceives Yoga merely as a beneficial movement and breathing practice. All the ancient verses are instructing Yoga; we just need to apply their instructions in our practice and teaching.

With more teaching experience, I became more skilful in integrating the ancient verses to my teaching. I started to run Yoga days for Yoga teachers with the title 'Integrating philosophy into general classes'. Those days were popular, and I was invited to teach them all over the UK. I learned that most Yoga teachers and practitioners have a yearning to find the 'philosophy' in their 'Yoga'. The more I taught the 'integration', the more I realized that I was trying to 'integrate Yoga into Yoga'. I don't use the term 'integrating' any more; I just teach the Indian tradition of Yoga. I study the ancient verses, let them teach me, experience their meaning in my practice and pass that experience on to my students.

The ancient verses are the source from which one can understand the practice of Yoga, including pranayama.

Pranayama is a process of controlling the pranic forces, which has always been taught throughout the history of Yoga and has been refined in the Hatha Yoga tradition. The understanding and practice of pranayama is clearly laid out in the Hatha verses. The most authoritative and inspiring Hatha composition is the Hatha Yoga Pradipika (HYP), allegedly composed by the sage Swatmarama in the 13th or 14th century CE. I learned to understand pranayama with the HYP in my hand.

Oral traditions that have been passed on for generations, like the HYP, have to be taken literally, and the Indian tradition is no exception. The Greek oral tradition we know as 'Homer' – the Iliad and Odyssey – was considered to be invented stories with no reliable historic base. Any attempt to find the remains of the city of Troy had failed, and Troy was therefore believed to have been a fiction invented by the composers of the Iliad. However, an early-20th-century German businessman, Heinrich Schliemann, believed in the historicity and reliability of the Homer verses. Following the geographical descriptions in the verses, he travelled to Turkey and found and excavated Troy (Vorphal 2019). In the same spirit, we have to take the HYP, follow it, practise it and find pranayama.

I can imagine the worried thoughts of some readers at this point, wondering whether the approach of following the old scriptures is not too regimented, causing us to lose our individuality and personal touch. We can develop our personal interpretation and style by following the original Yoga. Yoga is like music. To train to be a good musician, one cannot just sit in front of a piano and let creativity unfold. How can it unfold without any knowledge and skill? One needs to be taught by an expert, learn the notation system and principles of music harmony; one needs to train the fingers, learn to play scales…and then practise, practise, practise. When it comes to playing a skilful composition, such as a Beethoven sonata, a composition that instructs how every note is to be played – how long to hold it and how loud to play it – there seems to be no flexibility and personal expression, but there is. Those who can play every note at the right time and at the right volume differ enormously; they are very individual. Some do not excite their audience and some are world-class players who are loved and honoured. All have skill and knowledge, gained by strict instruction and practice, and on that basis they are able to be creative and express a personal touch and style.

In her book *Post-Lineage Yoga*, Theodora Wildcroft (2020) describes the differing personal approaches of the teachers she visited in her case studies. They vary widely, but they all had good basic training and developed their personal style from there.

The Indian masters did not teach stretching exercises to lengthen the hamstrings, they did not teach breathing exercises to increase lung capacity. They taught asana to free the blockages to get in touch with a deeper reality, and they taught pranayama, the method to free the subtle body from impurities, so that the aliveness within (Prana) can expand (ayama). The Indian masters did not teach relaxation. They taught meditation with the aim of Self-realization.

A different method: svadhyaya

Learning in the West used to be seen as a process of reading and studying, a process which is now rapidly changing in the digital era. To teach, we write books, and learning happens by reading the books. A non-fiction book is seen to be a construction of logically well-ordered information without repetition.

We wrongly assume that ancient India had the same learning

tradition of reading and studying books. Indian epics like the *Hitopadesha*, for example, classifiy people into those who are righteous and those who do not follow the dharma, are not generous and compassionate, and are 'andhigata shastra' – a term which is often translated to 'unread in the scriptures' (Sanskrit IGCSE 2019–2024).

There were no people 'well read' or 'unread' in the scriptures as there were no scriptures, just orally transmitted verses chanted by memory. The people praised in these stories had not read books, but rather memorized verses and chanted them repeatedly. This was the method of learning in ancient India, a method that is very effective. Rather than reading a text once and forgetting it, ongoing repetition allowed the teachings to become second nature. The lessons learned do not reside in the back of the brain, but they are present, lived. The Yoga Sutras of Patanjali describe this method as the fourth niyama in the eight limbs (the practices of Yoga), 'svadhyaya', which is often translated as 'study of the scriptures' but is actually meaning the practice of repeated chanting of the verses.

The folk song tradition in Europe worked in a similar way. Songs were repeatedly sung, and most songs had a refrain which brought the most important message back again and again, and everyone would remember it and join in singing.

I advise my Yoga teacher trainee students to constantly repeat the main message they want to bring across in a class, to create a lasting effect for their students. I use the analogy of a musical composition. A good composer is not one who invents as many tunes as possible for a piece, but one who has the skill to bring the same tune back again and again in different variations. A good composition will ensure the audience walks away from a performance humming the tune.

I try to adapt to the Indian learning method in this book by formulating a refrain-like statement, which is repeated frequently. Reading the statement might be confusing at first and the reader will soon have forgotten the wording, but I hope every repetition serves as a reminder, creates a better understanding and ingrains the message in the reader's mind.

This book is an attempt to stress and clarify these statements based on the evidence of the Sanskrit verses and decades of my own practice and teaching and learning Sanskrit.

Refrain

Pranayama is not respiration, but the expansion of Prana. Pranayama is a process not in the physical body but in the pranic body. Prana is not air or breath, but life that enters each embryo and settles in the navel centre; death occurs when Prana, life, leaves.

Pranayama, the expansion of Prana, is a threefold process: (1) the expanding of Prana from its origin in the navel centre outwards; (2) the reversing of Prana back to the navel centre; and (3) the containing of Prana in the navel centre. The threefold process is called vayu, and it happens in the rhythm of the breath, but it is not breath, and it moves in the opposite direction to respiration. Vayu does not move through air tubes but through nadis. The nadis are full of impurities, and pranayama is the purification process. Once the nadis are purified, the vayu stops moving and breath ceases. Prana then remains for prolonged periods in the navel centre where it creates heat, which awakens a dormant pranic force sitting in the base chakra, kundalini. Kundalini rises in the innermost, spiritual nadi, sushumna; when it reaches the top, sahasrara, an enlightened state occurs.

Chapter 1

SETTING THE SCENE

Yogis did not practise with their anatomical bodies

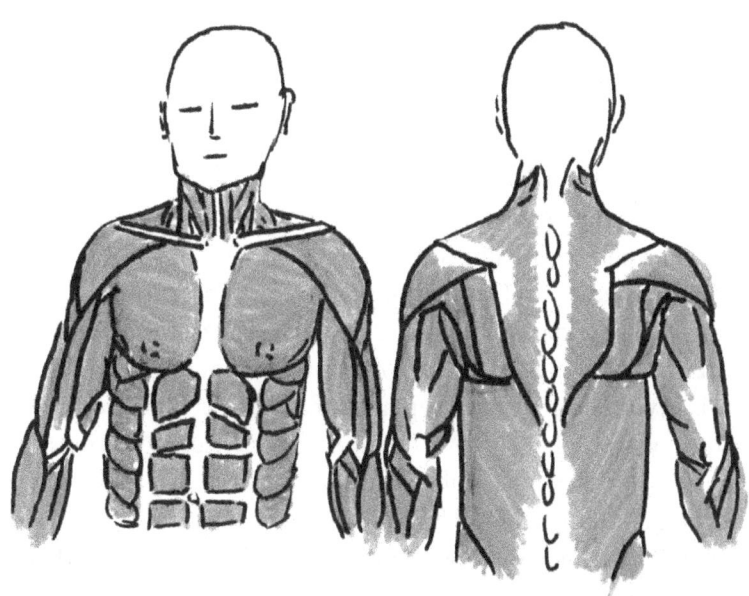

Figure 1.1 *The anatomical body*

What causes the trees to blossom in spring? How can chicks hatch from their eggs? A newborn baby is a miracle; what causes a child to grow, change from day to day, mature, age and eventually die? These are all signs of life. A living being is not a mechanical system, but a process. There is not a moment of stagnation; life forms are like clouds in permanent transformation. I found it an amazing experience watching my children grow up, an ever-changing process, in particular during their teenage years. Some days they left for school in the mornings, and upon returning home in the afternoon they had changed. One of my meditation teachers told us that he was looking at old photographs of his kids and was struck by the insight that the people in the pictures do not exist any more. His kids were certainly still alive, but they were not those people in the pictures. Humans are not static; life is not static. We are not mechanisms like clocks, often in need of repair, as the French philosopher René Descartes described us. Life is that which keeps us in permanent flux and flow. Life is a force within all living beings that changes and transforms us. This force is one of the most obvious phenomena but, ironically, we seem to overlook it. The Western mind tends to take snapshots of life and treat living beings as static things. When a human body is ailing, we change diseased parts like a clockmaker replaces worn-out gears. We do not reflect on the phenomenon of life, and we don't seem to notice that it is present within. We do not wonder why we are alive and what makes us so. We do not realize that life is a mystery, and we don't respect it. India has always respected and worshipped that phenomenon of life and named it 'Prana'.

Prana is life force, aliveness; ayama is expansion. Pranayama therefore is the expansion of aliveness in the bodily system.

Modern medics understand the 'bodily system' in terms of static anatomy and physiology. Western science has made enormous progress in understanding and treating the human anatomy, saving many lives. There is nevertheless a non-acceptance of any aspect of humanity other than the anatomical reality. Western medical science, and with it a large proportion of the general public, attempts to find all forms of human expression in the anatomical body. If human expressions such as aliveness, life (Prana) and consciousness do not fit into the model, they are not believed to exist or are just not seen.

The anatomical body consists of different systems working together: the hard inner frame – the skeletal system; the soft tissue moving the bones – the muscular system; the transport of nutrition and oxygen – the cardiovascular system; the communication structures passing information between the systems – the nervous and endocrine systems; and the processes of bringing the building blocks for the body from the outside into the body – the digestive and the respiratory systems. All those systems are well researched and can be effectively treated when a dysfunction occurs. That approach uses perceiving with our five senses and investigating under a microscope:

> Current science usually starts from a reality that is based solely on perceptible phenomena. (Van Lommel 2010, p.xvi)

There is more to us than perceptible phenomena. The more we learn about the anatomical aspects of the human body, the more we should be amazed. All these systems cooperate in an unimaginably complex way, and they usually function perfectly. We are so focused on understanding *how* it all works that we forget to see *why* it all works: we do not see the wood for the trees. We overlook the fact that the system is alive and that there is an amazing intelligence keeping the anatomy going; there is consciousness within, awareness, being able to experience, being a witness of the world around us.

Aspects like life and consciousness and many others do obviously exist, but medical science has either overlooked them or unsuccessfully attempted to locate these phenomena in the human anatomy.

Consciousness is not an anatomical process

We are conscious; there is no question of that. Believing that human existence is merely an anatomical process must raise the question 'Where is consciousness located in the body?' We tend to look for it in the brain, not because there is clear evidence of consciousness being in the brain, but it seems implausible to look for consciousness in other parts such as bones or muscles. The materialistic, scientific approach 'is based on the premise that consciousness is a product or effect of brain function… The approach is generally not made explicit and simply taken for granted without any kind of debate' (van Lommel 2010, p.243).

Van Lommel, quoted above, is a Dutch cardiologist and a researcher of near-death experience (NDE). He and many others have collected thousands of reports of people who had clear, conscious experiences in a state where their brain was dead. Experiences of this kind have been recorded for millennia. They have always occurred, but they are becoming much more common since we have had effective methods of resuscitation. These experiences are often classified as false anecdotes in the belief that it is not be possible to be conscious with a non-functioning brain. But it apparently is: these experiences exist, and we shouldn't conjure them away just because they do not fit into our belief systems. Consciousness is not a brain function, and no one has ever found consciousness in the brain. Consciousness is a non-anatomical entity; it does not sit in the brain or anywhere else in the human anatomy and physiology. It is not of material substance and is not locatable:

> I strongly believe that consciousness cannot be located in a particular time and place. This is known as nonlocality. Complete and endless consciousness is everywhere in a dimension that is not tied to time or place, where past, present, and future all exist and are accessible at the same time. (Van Lommel 2010, p.xvii)

What the Dutch cardiologist expresses here should sound familiar to every practitioner who has taken an interest in the spiritual side of Yoga. A consciousness that is endless, not locatable, of no size and physical attributes, was the main topic of the old Indian seekers sitting in isolation in the forests and meditating. Their teaching was collected in the compositions called the Upanishads.

> It [consciousness, Self, Atman] is neither big nor small, neither long nor short, neither hot nor cold, neither bright nor dark, neither air nor space. It is without attachment, without taste, smell or touch, without eyes, ears, tongue, mouth, breath, or mind, without movement, without limitations, without inside or outside. It consumes nothing, and nothing is consuming it. (Easwaran 1988, chapter III, 7–8)

Consciousness, Atman or Purusha in Sanskrit, cannot be discovered by research or thought: 'thoughts can never reach it' (Easwaran 1988, Taittiriya Upanishad II, 9), but thought-free introspection, which is called meditation, can realize it, in a process that transcends physicality. The Yogis did not meditate with their bodies.

Life is not an anatomical process

There is no question that we are alive. There is a difference between a body that is alive and one that is dead. The organs and the brain in a living body work; when they stop working, the body is dead, but that does not explain the phenomenon of life. Organs in a living body work; they stop working when life departs. The reason the organs and the brain work is that they are empowered by a subtle force, Prana. A hairdryer works when empowered by electricity and ceases to function when electricity 'leave' – it is merely a construction of metal and plastic. Likewise, a body is a mere mass of organic material when Prana leaves. Prana, which is of a more subtle nature than electricity, departing causes the brain and all other organs to cease to function; life is gone, and the body is dead.

Life is the phenomenon which keeps each living creature in permanent change. Life is the phenomenon that leaves when death occurs, and it is called Prana by the ancient Yogis.

Grasping the phenomenon of Prana is difficult with a Western upbringing. In my 20 years of training Yoga teachers, I found that course participants had no problem writing essays on muscular analysis, Patanjali, pranayama, chakras or nadi, but the essay topic 'Prana' was the one they found very difficult.

Prana cannot be seen under a microscope, but when turning inwards with a still mind – in other words, when we meditate – we 'see' our aliveness. The Prashna Upanishad talks about seekers who gained understanding of life in the process of meditation.

Four seekers leave their worldly life behind and move into the forest to find the sage Pippalada dwelling in the forest in isolation. They asked him for teachings. Pippalada did not instruct them to sit down and listen to his wisdom, but he asked them to live with him for a year and meditate for questions to arise. An answer is only of value when a question precedes it. Sitting in meditation opened the seekers' minds and they began to wonder, 'What is this life within me and all other beings?' After the first year of meditation, one of the seekers uttered the question: 'Master, who created the universe?' (Easwaran 1988, Prashna Upanishad, Question I, 3). The master answered: 'The Lord meditated and brought forth prana' (Easwaran 1988, Prashna Upanishad, Question I, 4). The answer was not: God created the land, water and animals and humans, but the Divine created Prana, life.

After another year of meditation passed, the seekers formulated the question: 'Master, what powers support this body?' (Easwaran 1988, Prashna Upanishad, Question II, 1) There is life, Prana – how does it stand in relationship with other elements? To answer this question, Pippalada related an anecdote. All physical organs and elements of the body debate who the most important is. Prana convinces all physical functions that they cannot exist without Prana: 'To demonstrate the truth, prana rose and left the body, and all the powers knew they had to leave as well. When prana returned to the body, they too were back.' (Easwaran 1988, Prashna Upanishad, Question II, 4).

It is life that holds a body together, and this life is not an anatomical process but the basis of all existence.

Pranayama is not an anatomical process

Pranayama is not a physical practice. Defining pranayama using anatomical language does not do it justice.

Because the West perceives the human phenomenon solely as an anatomical process, Yoga has changed since being introduced in the West. Yoga was adjusted to Western views and defined using anatomical terminology. The Hatha Yoga tradition does not use anatomical terms, however. Pranayama is described as a movement (vayu) of life (Prana) in subtle conductors (nadis), none of which are locatable in the anatomical body.

It is commonly assumed that Prana is 'breath' because there is a Prana-breath link, and life starts with the first breath and ends with the last. But I believe that the identification of pranayama with respiration is incorrect.

The first Westerner to write a book with the title *Pranayama* was André Van Lysebeth (1919–2004), a Belgian Yoga instructor and author who helped to make Yoga popular in Europe by publishing books that have been translated into many languages. In his book *Pranayama: The Yoga of Breathing* (1972), Van Lysebeth respects the Indian tradition, and he saw in Prana more than just breath. He understood that the Yoga tradition referred to a more complex process, but he tried to express his view in Western terms. He took the view that Prana is vitalizing ions in the air. He equated Prana with electricity and therefore thought it would be used up and that we are in permanent need of recharging. He thought that pranic particles are in the air and enter the human system via breath, or via skin and food.

> Several thousands of years before our scientists identified electricity the yogis had revealed that the atmosphere vibrates with a subtle energy and that this energy is the main source of all kinds of energy active in the human body. (Lysbeth 1972, p.8)

Prana is not electricity: a computer, a vacuum cleaner and a hairdryer run on electricity, but they are not alive.

Following Van Lysebeth's definition, Prana was equated with 'energy', which does not match the yogic meaning. Energy is used up, but Prana resides in a body from conception to death.

All life is an expression of Prana, not just humans and animals who are breathing. Non-respiring life such as plants are also alive by the presence of Prana.

Van Lysebeth saw himself that the Indian conception was a more subtle process, but maintained the scientific view:

> To interpret pranayama as breathing exercise would be to limit sadly the scope of the exercises and to misunderstand their true purpose, which is the collecting, storing and conscious control of the vital pranic energies in our bodies. (Van Lysebeth 1972, p.6)

Whatever Van Lysebeth means by these words 'Prana does not move in our bodies but in nadis'.

The nadis are the 'place' where pranayama occurs. The nadis are a network of subtle conductors of the pranic life force penetrating not the physical body but an invisible, intangible reality beyond the physical. When the concept of nadis became known in the West, the nadis were sought within human anatomy. There are conductors penetrating the anatomical system – the nerves – which led to the conclusion that nadis are nerves; they certainly are not, even though we still find 20th-century Yoga books using the term 'nerves' when referring to nadis.

The Hatha Yoga Pradipika and other Hatha verses explain clearly what pranayama is; we just need to engage with it. Instead of looking at the old Hatha verses, the West attempted to explain pranayama with contemporary Western science.

Pranayama is not a process that can be seen and studied, it is an inner experience, taking place in a dimension that the outer five senses and thought cannot reach. Pranayama is not a breathing exercise, despite the fact that aspects of the pranayama process are linked to the breath.

Refrain

Pranayama is not respiration, but the expansion of Prana. Pranayama is a process not in the physical body but in the pranic body. Prana is not air or breath, but life that enters each embryo and settles in the navel centre; death occurs when Prana, life, leaves.

Pranayama, the expansion of Prana, is a threefold process: (1) the expanding of Prana from its origin in the navel centre outwards; (2) the reversing of Prana back to the navel centre; and (3) the containing of Prana in the navel centre. The threefold process is called vayu, and it happens in the rhythm of the breath, but it is not breath, and it moves in the opposite direction to respiration. Vayu does not move through air tubes but through nadis. The nadis are full of impurities, and pranayama is the purification process. Once the nadis are purified, the vayu stops moving and breath ceases. Prana then remains for prolonged periods in the navel centre where it creates heat, which awakens a dormant pranic force sitting in the base chakra, kundalini. Kundalini rises in the innermost, spiritual nadi, sushumna; when it reaches the top, sahasrara, an enlightened state occurs.

Indian medical science did not work with the anatomical body

India has, unlike the West, never seen human life as a purely anatomical process. Anatomy was never an important topic in Indian culture. India had, and still has, a very refined and advanced medical healing system – Ayurveda – which is based on Yoga 'philosophy'. Ayurveda does not describe human nature as a composition of bones, muscles and organs. It does not divide the human body into categories of systems such as cardiovascular, nervous and respiratory. Ayurveda sees a human as a product of their lifestyle and a play of different components (guna), activity and creativity (rajas), lethargy and destruction (tamas), and illumination and transcendence (sattvas). Humans come in different dominances or body types (doshas): lightness, the element air (vata); creativity, stability and fire (pitta); and being grounded, heaviness, slowness (kapha). Bodies are a combination of different layers (koshas – see below). Ayurveda treats non-anatomical aspects; lost balance of the mentioned elements is restored, and all aspects are brought into harmony. Ayurveda has been around for thousands of years, and it is still practised today, which in itself is proof of its value. People have benefitted from Ayurveda for a long time. Ayurveda has never entered the Western mainstream as it does not fulfil our norms; its benefits cannot be explained on the anatomical level, and it has therefore been classified as ineffective.

Yoga works on deeper, non-physical dimensions

The Western view that we are a sole anatomical body, and that all human aspects are explicable from that point of view, is new. In the past, there was a clear understanding of a non-physical entity within us – the soul – which is temporarily linked to the body and then moves on after death. Many cultures are familiar with this phenomenon – from Islam to Buddhism, to Hinduism, Shamanism and Christianity. As modern science has concluded that our anatomical knowledge is so all-compassing that we can explain all human expressions with it, we have come to reject different contemporary cultures and those of other times. But other cultures have come to knowledge and understanding by searching in non-anatomical realms that can be experienced, and their results have to be taken as seriously.

Indian culture has understood, throughout time, that the core of each human, the inner essence, is consciousness, Self (with a capital S), the entity within us that experiences. Our true Self is not the body, not our individuality, not our Ego and not our history, but a non-locatable and unchanging consciousness (see the section above, 'Consciousness is not an anatomical process') – what still exists after the death of the body. This entity has attached itself to a physicality. A physicality that is not the one body, but interwoven layers of different densities, from gross to subtle to even more subtle. Consciousness itself has no density or substance; it stays connected for the duration of life not just to one body, but to five, called 'koshas' (sheaths, layer). They are:

- **Annamaya kosha** (anna = food; maya = made of) is the visible body, made out of food. This is the anatomical body our culture is familiar with. We have access to this body via our five senses.

- **Pranamaya kosha** is the body made of Prana, the 'aliveness' body with all its vayus (winds), chakras (whirly condensed pranic centres), nadis, granthis and malas (subtle obstructions in the pranic body). We have access to the pranic body through an inner direct perception; the pranic body is what we perceive when we turn our awareness inwards.
- **Manomaya kosha** (manas = mind) is the body of thought and attachment. Mind is not located in the brain. The physical brain only displays the mind's activities like a TV screen; the program is not contained in the physical TV device. Yogis speak about a space outside of the physical body, about two and a half inches in front of the point between our eyebrows, where mental imaging takes place. This is known as the drishti space, and images sit here and not in the brain. The mind is a realm on its own. To clear and empty the mind space is the process of Yoga. In contrast to our understanding, Yoga 'philosophy' does not mention positive thoughts, feelings and emotions, only thoughts and attachments which are all obstacles to human development. Feelings and emotions are fluctuating experiences which come and go; they are classified in Yoga 'philosophy' as attachments which need to be overcome. Yoga exploration differentiates inner processes in great detail. What seems likeable might not be as positive as we tend to believe. For example, we chase after entertainment or possessions thinking they make us happy, but the sensation when those are attained is not happiness, but just satisfaction of a craving. We say we love someone, without being aware that the underlying sensation might be a need, an attachment, not love and happiness. Attachments are movements, (vrittis) in manomaya kosha, and as such cover up the deeper layers and therefore are all 'negative' obstacles. The deeper koshas (vijnanamaya kosha and anandamaya kosha) accommodate happiness, love and insight, which are not emotions but inert properties, always present in full form. Happiness, love and insight are rooted in the deeper bodies, are covered by impurities, thoughts and attachments, and are experienced when inner clarity and stillness occurs, not as a result of outer circumstances. This is an important fact to be aware of when working with pranayama. All koshas are interwoven, and attachments formed in the mind

space leave impurities in the pranamaya kosha, which can be freed by the practice of pranayama. Thought processes happen at all times; most of them happen unconsciously. They stimulate each other and are often in overdrive and out of control.

- **Vijnanamaya kosha** (vi = down, into; jnana = wisdom) is the space of inner knowledge, insight, jnana. Insight is present by nature; it does not need to be taught or learned. The West understands learning as a process from the outside to the inside, knowledge being uploaded into our memories. The East has found a different way, namely turning inwards and reaching through the busy thought layers to the inner wisdom, which does not come from the outside in, but from the inside out.
- **Anandamaya kosha** (ananda = bliss) is the deepest layer. When clearing the physical body of toxins and tensions, the pranic body of impurities, the mental body of thoughts and attachments, and activating the inner wisdom, the deepest layer can be reached – a blissful state. The more transparent our koshas become, the happier we are. Unhappiness results from blocked koshas, not from outer circumstances.

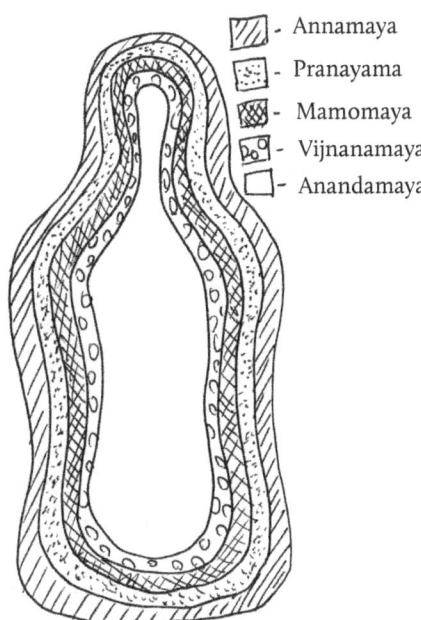

Figure 1.2 *The koshas – the five sheaths of the human bodily system*

The division of the human body into five koshas or layers is first mentioned in the Taittiriya Upanishad. It has been known throughout the history of Yoga and has been refined by Ayurveda, Tantra and Hatha.

Yoga has never emphasized work on the anatomical body, annamaya kosha. The Hatha repertoire of practices contains: shatkarma (preliminary cleansing), asana (postures), pranayama (leave untranslated to avoid misinterpretation), mudras (gestures) and concentration on nada (inner sound), all with the aim to attain 'unmani', the perfected, enlightened state, reaching the Self beyond the koshas.

Shatkarma works on the physical level, but is seen as preliminary to Yoga practice. The shatkarmas remove phlegm and mucus, but are also practised to balance the three humours (doshas) (HYP 2, 21). Asana is seen as the first step in the Hatha practice sequence:

> Asana creates steadiness, health and lightness of body. (HYP 1, 17)

Asana practice undoubtedly results in physical benefits and freedom from maladies, but the main purpose is gaining awareness of obstructions and impurities in the pranic kosha. Physical benefits, though not only physical benefits, are mentioned:

> Pashcimatana [seated forward bend] is splendid, it makes the wind [pavan, synonym to vayu] flow in the west [the back, here sushumna]; it increases the fire of the belly, makes the abdomen small and brings health to men. (HYP 1, 29)

Pranayama is the method of clearing the obstruction and impurities from pranamaya kosha.

Mudras come in the form of eye and tongue movements, whole-body practices and bandhas (see Chapter 5 in this book). They do not result in physical benefits:

> Therefore, with all effort [practise mudras] to awaken the Goddess [kundalini], sleeping at the door of Brahman. (HYP 3, 5)

Mudras are thus also working in the field of pranamaya kosha.

In nada practice, one connects to internal sounds, waves of non-material substance. The focus is turned inwards and sharpened so that nada can be heard, which helps to loosen obstructions, granthis, in pranamaya kosha (HYP 94, 69). This shows that...

Hatha Yoga works with the pranic and not the physical body.

All the Hatha practices are steps to 'attain the superior Raja-Yoga [the state of still mind]' (HYP 1,1).

The 1500-year-old Raja Yoga tradition, which we know from the Yoga Sutras of Patanjali, works on manomaya kosha, stilling the mind for deeper layers to become activated. Raja Yoga is defined as 'Yogah citta [mind space] vritti [movement, activity] nirodha [cessation]' (Patanjali 1, 2).

Raja Yoga works on the mental, manomaya, not the physical body.

The Karma Yoga tradition of the Bhagavad Gita works on manomaya kosha, the ultimate detachment process. Bhakti Yoga, as instructed in the Bhagavad Gita and the Upanishads, reaches into anandamaya kosha, and the Jnana Yoga of the Upanishads operates on vijnanamaya kosha. No Yoga tradition has the physical body, annamaya kosha, as its field of action.

Refrain

Pranayama is not respiration, but the expansion of Prana. Pranayama is a process not in the physical body but in the pranic body. Prana is not air or breath, but life that enters each embryo and settles in the navel centre; death occurs when Prana, life, leaves.

Pranayama, the expansion of Prana, is a threefold process: (1) the expanding of Prana from its origin in the navel centre outwards; (2) the reversing of Prana back to the navel centre; and (3) the containing of Prana in the navel centre. The threefold process is called vayu, and it happens in the rhythm of the breath, but it is not breath, and it moves in the opposite direction to respiration. Vayu does not move through air tubes but through nadis. 'The nadis are full of impurities' (HYP 2, 3), and pranayama is the purification process. Once the nadis are purified, the vayu stops moving and breath ceases. Prana then remains for prolonged periods in the navel centre where it creates heat, which awakens a dormant pranic force sitting in the base chakra, kundalini. Kundalini rises in the innermost, spiritual nadi, sushumna; when it reaches the top, sahasrara, an enlightened state occurs.

Chapter 2

HATHA YOGA – THE TRADITION THAT REFINED PRANAYAMA

The concept of Prana up to the Hatha times

Prana is defined as 'the principle of vitality in the individual organism, whereby it is said to be all-pervading, invisible, and the life duration of all' (Grimes 1996).

Most Yoga concepts go back thousands of years to the Vedas which are Yoga's major building blocks, its bricks. **The Vedas**, which means 'knowledge' in Sanskrit, are oral traditions, poetic verses which originated possibly more than 5000 years ago. They are seen as sacred, timeless, without an author. The Indian tradition refers to their originator with the term 'Vyasa'. It is often said that Vyasa is the name of the author, but Vyasa means 'compiler'; the Vedas are a process rather than the work of a specific person. All 'houses' throughout the history of Yoga were built with the 'bricks' from the Vedas.

The earliest evidence of the concept of Prana can be found in the Rig Veda, where it is described as the phenomenon of life. Prana is everything that gives life, the breath, the sun, water, as stated in the Atharvaveda:

> When Prana showered with torrents of rain on the great earth, then all living beings rejoice: there is going to be great plenty of food and prosperity, they celebrate. When showered over and regaled, herbs and trees speak to Prana together: 'You have given us life and more, you have given us all the beauty and fragrance of life'. (11.4, 5-6)

The Upanishads give the first structured concept of Prana. The Prashna

Upanishad defines Prana as the first creation of the Divine: first there was life and only then did life enter into different life forms.

> Prana is born of the Self (divine consciousness). As a man casts a shadow, the Self casts prana into the body at the time of birth. (Easwaran 1988: Prashna Upanishad, Question II, 3)

One of the first mentions of the subdivision of Prana into the vayus (winds) – prana, apana, samana, vyana, udana – is found in the Prashna Upanishad. This division becomes an important feature in the later Hatha tradition.

In classical Yoga, the Yoga Sutras of Patanjali do not emphasize Prana. Patanjali works with mind control. Pranayama is nevertheless listed as one of the main practices, the third of the eight limbs (Patanjali 2, 50–52). The vayus are not taught, but the knowledge of the Prana subdivision of vayu is apparent in the third chapter. Verse 40 instructs focus on udana to become able to levitate, and verse 41 instructs focus on samana to become radiant in body.

The 'Prana bricks' from the Vedas and Upanishads are much later picked up by **Tantra** and a solid house is built. Tantra also refined the concept of the human koshas from the Taittiriya Upanishad (Easwaran 1988: Taittiriya Upanishad II, 2.1–6.1). We are Consciousness, Self, Atman, which expresses itself in this lifetime in the form of a five-layered body, pancha (five) kosha (see the section 'Yoga works on deeper, non-physical dimensions' in Chapter 1). Tantra explored the subtler, deeper, unsubstantial layer of pranayama kosha, where Prana moves (vayu) in specific pathways (nadis); the sheath made out of Prana is not detectable with the senses and cannot seen under a microscope.

The Tantra tradition explored and experienced pranamaya kosha in detail. The Tantrists' insights were adopted by the Hatha tradition, starting to form in the fifth century CE. The great achievement of Hatha Yoga was to find methods and practices which enable the practitioner to manipulate that pranic sheath. Life – Prana – is there as long as we live – we do not need to replenish or increase it – but if that sheath of Prana is blocked, a method is needed to unblock the sheath, a method to expand (ayama) Prana – a method called pranayama.

Prana is the 'Hatha Yoga anatomy'

Hatha is the school of Yoga which worked predominantly with the pranamaya kosha, the sheath made of Prana, the life within. Most people in the West who have some idea about Yoga know the term Hatha Yoga, but no one seems to know what Hatha really is. Some schools of Yoga in the West have clear definitions: there is Ashtanga Yoga, three sequences of strenuous asana composed by Pathabi Jois; there is Iyengar Yoga, a very detailed, focused asana work devised by B.K.S. Iyengar; there is Bikram Yoga or hot Yoga, a sequence practised in a very hot room taught by Bikram Choudhury; there is Vinyasa flow, which is a modern form of movement using asana not in the original still form but in flowing movement…and there are many Yoga classes that don't fall under any of those categories. In the absence of a category, the latter are usually referred to as 'Hatha Yoga', an arbitrary classification. Hatha has lost its original meaning.

> Curiously, in the last dozen years, hatha yoga has somehow come to refer to a style of practising asana, instead of a wide range of practices including pranayama, cleansing practices, bandhas, mudras, all asanas and more. It reminds me of the telephone game where a whispered message goes from ear to ear around the room, to the amusement of all when the last message is compared with the original. Perhaps it is time to hear from the original sources of hatha yoga and set the record straight. (Anderson 2017)

Hatha Yoga has changed in the West, as if in a game of Chinese whispers. The process of change is hardly noticeable, but comparing the end result with the original Indian tradition is astonishing.

Hatha worked with the pranic body, pranamaya kosha; it is a subtle invisible reality that cannot be seen, cannot be touched, but can be experienced.

It is actually the pranic body and not the anatomical body we experience when we turn our senses to the inner space. When we apply a still posture and turn awareness inwards, without the use of the five senses or thought processes distracting us, we experience 'the within'. This experience 'within' is not bones, muscles or organs; the process of digestion in the stomach and guts cannot be felt, nor the circulation of the blood or the detoxing of the liver. We have no direct experience of our anatomical body.

We cannot even feel the shape and form of the body. When muscles are relaxed during a good Yoga practice, then there is no perception of the physical form. All practitioners love that state where the physical body 'disappears', but we don't tend to reflect on what that means: we cannot perceive the anatomical body directly, but we do perceive and enjoy something – there is something other.

The exploration of that which can be perceived is the 'Hatha Yoga science'. Bright and alive areas can be felt; others are dull. Some inner places stand out; others are unaware. Those that stand out are not of substance, are not tangible, have no material substance; they are more like sensations and qualities. We also feel resistances, clinging, holding on, which is not tightness of muscles – we cannot feel muscles. The shape of this experienced space seems not to be defined; it can widen and shrink. A rhythmical movement from somewhere in the middle of that experienced space is perceived, outwards and reversing back, an expanding of aliveness. This movement is not respiration, although we believe it is, because it shares the same rhythm as respiration; we believe it because we have no concept of any perceptible rhythmical movement other than respiration.

What we feel is not air flowing through the nostrils into the lungs, but a very slow, pulsating movement somewhere well below the respiratory system in the area where the abdomen is located in the physical body.

The Hatha Yogis gave these sensations of aliveness various names: the rhythmical movement from the navel centre was called vayu (wind); the areas where aliveness moves were called nadi (conductor); bright centres were called chakra (wheel); clinging and blocked areas were called granthi (knot) or mala kulasa (obstacles clinging on). We could, like the Hatha Yogis, gain complete knowledge of the pranayama kosha, but two factors prevent this.

First, our knowledge. When we sit still and close our eyes, we have no direct experience of the physical, but only knowledge and memory of it. This tricks us, and we cannot isolate knowledge from direct experience. We have an inner vision of sitting upright, with legs and arms and a head, as a physical body.

When applying asana, we feel blocked areas that cling, and we assume we feel tight muscles, because we are taught to expect only muscles in these areas. We cannot feel muscles but the obstacles that block and cling in pranamaya kosha and prevent Prana from expanding. When we release the blocking and clinging, Prana expands and we feel aliveness – nothing else, not muscles.

Second, our direct experience cannot perceive much as long as the pranic body is full of obstructions. In an obstructed pranamaya kosha, there is not much Prana moving, and as such there is no 'aliveness' and awareness; areas with low-level Prana are not felt. After a good, releasing Yoga practice, it is easier to perceive and explore the inner space.

Having instructed students in a Yoga class to directly perceive, I pointed out that we cannot feel the anatomical body parts. One woman laughed and said, 'Certainly, we do not feel our bones and muscles.' We know this, our life experience tells us this, so why do we not reflect what it actually is that we sense and why don't we question why we do not feel the body we believe we are feeling? We are programmed to believe that all there is to us is our anatomy; anything else is a subjective feeling not to be taken seriously. The Hatha Yogis took these 'subjective feelings' seriously and created a science and a practice based on the invisible, untouchable realm, pranamaya kosha.

The rhythmical movement we feel is a subtle expanding of awareness, lightness, aliveness, Prana, establishing a pranic field, pranamaya kosha. The outwards expansion could continue for a long time, reaching throughout the whole of the inner space, but it does not; something blocks it. After the expansion, the awareness, lightness, aliveness, Prana reverses back into the navel centre, which can also be a very prolonged process, although it is usually not. The flow is blocked. The reverse can be followed by a moment of stillness, but usually the stillness is broken. By sharpening the focus on pranic movement, the nature of the obstructions becomes more obvious. Some of the inner space is impenetrable. This experience was formulated by the Hatha Yogis with the words 'the nadis are full of impurities' (HYP 2, 3). Free from anatomical programming, the Yogis perceived that Prana has its origin in the area of the navel centre. The expanding force does not move through the nostrils and air tubes and lungs; it moves through a subtle network of nadis covering the whole of the inner space. The subtle movement becomes obvious when one has overcome the anatomical programming.

When I instructed a new group of students in pranayama recently, one woman said, 'I call this diaphragmatic breath.' However, it is not: diaphragmatic breath causes the diaphragm to contract and compress the abdominal organs during an inhalation. The sensation of pranayama during an inhalation is that of expanding and not compressing. In diaphragmatic respiration, an element moves inwards – that is why we call it inhalation. The pranic expansion is an outwards movement. Exhalation, on the other hand, starts with high pressure in the lungs, which then lessens, causing the exhalation to start strong, getting weaker and eventually petering out, like deflating a rubber dinghy. The sensation of pranayama during the exhalation is the return of life to the navel centre. Exhalation is an outward movement; the return of Prana is an inward movement. It is the power of the navel centre that draws the Prana back, in the way that a black hole sucks galaxies inward, and as such the reverse increases in strength and does not peter out.

The ironic fact is that lots of Yoga practitioners and teachers learn about the pranic elements – the vayus, nadis, granthis and chakras and the description of pranayama. But when it comes to practice, the physical body moves into postures and the breath flows in and out of the lungs. When the pranic process is not experienced, all knowledge of Prana, nadis, chakras and vayus remains theoretical and as such is useless. I always tell my students that the Hatha Yogis did not construct a clever system, but they sat, practised and experienced and formulated their experience for us, so that we can recreate the same experience in our practice.

When we believe that the rhythmical movement within is physical respiration and nothing more, then we will miss the pranic experience – we see only what we expect.

We believe that what we can't see or pick up with our outer senses does not exist and therefore we do not register even the clearest and most obvious pranic sensation.

Refrain

Pranayama is not respiration, but the expansion of Prana. Pranayama is a process not in the physical body but in the pranic body. Prana is not air or breath, but life that enters each embryo and settles in the navel centre; death occurs when Prana, life, leaves.

Pranayama, the expansion of Prana, is a threefold process: (1) the expanding of Prana from its origin in the navel centre outwards; (2) the reversing of Prana back to the navel centre; and (3) the containing of Prana in the navel centre. The threefold process is called vayu, and it happens in the rhythm of the breath, but it is not breath, and it moves in the opposite direction to respiration. Vayu does not move through air tubes but through nadis. The nadis are full of impurities, and pranayama is the purification process. Once the nadis are purified, the vayu stops moving and breath ceases. Prana then remains for prolonged periods in the navel centre where it creates heat, which awakens a dormant pranic force sitting in the base chakra, kundalini. Kundalini rises in the innermost, spiritual nadi, sushumna; when it reaches the top, sahasrara, an enlightened state occurs.

The historical journey of pranayama from Hatha to modern Yoga

Prana and pranayama were topics predominantly dealt with in Hatha Yoga, the Yoga of Ha (sun – the main nadi sightly left of centre, often referred to with the term 'ida') and Tha (moon, the main nadi slightly right of centre, often referred to with the term 'pingala'), the Yoga working with pranamaya kosha.

The Hatha practice flourished from around 400 CE to 1800 CE, up to the time of the British Empire. The British arrived in India for trading in 1608 and started invading in 1757; in 1857, the British Crown officially took control of the whole of the Indian subcontinent. At that time, India was a highly cultured and wealthy country, and the cultural tradition was transmitted on a purely oral basis. The Vedas, Upanishads, Darshana and Hatha compositions were passed on unchanged from generation to generation for centuries. The wisdom was chanted, and the culture was practised. This way of learning was very foreign to the British, and therefore it was not promoted, resulting in the near extinction of the Hatha tradition and teaching. The only compositions that survived were those that had been put in writing.

B.K.S. Iyengar reported that it was barely possible in his youth to find a Hatha teacher. The British, showing an interest in Yoga, made it an academic subject at their newly founded Indian universities. Under British rule, academic teaching, hitherto unknown in India, became the way of learning. Indian learning changed from oral transmission and practice to academic study. The ten top Indian universities were founded between 1818 and 1916, with three of them, Kolkata, Mumbai and Chennai, founded in 1857, the year of the official takeover by the British.

Krishnamacharya, one of the greatest Yoga figures in the 20th century, trained teachers to bring Yoga to the West. Born in 1888, he wanted to learn Yoga and undertook the only path available at the time – university degrees. He achieved six degrees on all six darshanas (the six 'philosophical' schools from around 500–300 BCE) and realized that Yoga cannot be leaned as an academic subject. Subsequently, he walked all the way to the mountains in Tibet to one of the remaining authentic teachers, Yogeshwara Ramamohana Bramacharia, and lived with him for seven years. This teacher taught him and instructed the oral composition of the **Yoga Kurantha**. Krishnamacharya claimed that all he ever taught came from the Yoga Kurantha, a very asana-based style of teaching. His statement was doubted because no one ever found the Yoga Kurantha. No one could: the Yoga Kurantha was never written down, following the Indian way of oral transmission. The Yoga Kurantha was lost after Krishnamachaya's death; he was the last person to have memorized it and he did not pass the verses on to his students, only the postures. The four most influential students of Krishnamacharya were his son T.K.V. Desikachar, Pathabi Jois, B.K.S. Iyengar and Indra Devi. They introduced asana-based Yoga to the West. Western Yoga is therefore based on the Yoga Kurantha, not on Hatha Yoga.

Those Hatha compositions that had found written form were translated into European languages in the second half of the 20th century. The translators approached them with a Western mindset. Every translation is an interpretation, and the Hatha tradition was translated and interpreted in a Western way. The need to discover the real Hatha Yoga became apparent at the beginning of the 21st century. The London university SOAS (School of Oriental and African Studies) received a grant to run the Hatha Yoga Project from 2015 to 2020. This was the first attempt to discover the real Hatha. The project revealed that very little is known of the original Hatha Yoga, recorded in old Sanskrit scriptures and manuscripts.

Lost in translation

Hatha Yoga methods have been developed by Yogis in practice, not by sitting at a desk and writing, nor by pondering or the use of the five senses. Yogis followed a tradition that is thousands of years old, a tradition that was experimental, a tradition that saw a higher level of truth in experience than in outer appearance, a tradition which defined jnana (direct perception) as the path to truth rather than pramana (knowledge gained by the five senses, inference and testimony; Patanjali 1, 7).

Western culture studied the human body with a microscope and discovered details of human anatomy, but the Yogis studied the human make-up by sitting and directly perceiving. They perceived Prana and its movement (vayu) in pathways (nadis), they experienced spaces of whirling aliveness with different qualities (chakras), they experienced tendencies of holding and clinging (malas) and dense, impenetrable areas (granthis). Western scholars discovered a central structure in the body, the spine and spinal cord. Yogis experienced a centre of aliveness in the core of the human system, which can be awakened by practice (sushumna).

When translating old Hatha verses into European languages, there were no words for the Yogis' experiences. English anatomical terms were used for translations. The terms 'Prana' and 'vayu' were translated as the English word 'breath', which is a term associated with physical respiration. 'Pranayama' was translated as 'breathing practice', 'nadi' as 'nerves' and 'sushumna' as 'spine', and 'ida' and 'pingala' (the two sides of the nadis system right and left of sushumna) were translated as 'right or left nostril'. The reader of these translations is unknowingly guided towards an anatomical understanding, away from the Yogis' experience. For some of the Yogis' terms, no Western substitutes were found – for example, for the words 'kundalini' (the dormant power sitting in the lowest chakra) or 'bindu' (the source of creational power at the back of the head) or 'nada' (internal sounds from a subtle plane heard in concentration). These words were left untranslated, creating a bizarre mix of health-promoting exercises and esoteric weirdness. This bizarre mix might very well be the main reason that the Western world has disregarded Hatha compositions as reliable sources. Compositions like Patanjali, the Upanishads and the Bhagavad Gita were instantly loved in the West, because they describe practices on the mental, ethical and spirit planes, which are familiar to us.

When the Hatha Yoga Pradipika (HYP) was taught when I trained to become a Yoga teacher, 30 years ago, we were advised to 'take it with a pinch of salt'. No one would give this advice when studying the Bhagavad Gita, that would be inappropriate. I believe that it is in the same way inappropriate to advise readers of the HYP to 'take the teaching with a pinch of salt', because the Yogis had a reason for every word. Imagine if we have not studied mathematics in school and someone asks us to read a mathematical article. We would not take the article with a pinch of salt; we have to learn the language of mathematics to understand it. Our lack of prior knowledge would not invalidate the mathematical article, and, in the same way, our lack of prior knowledge should not invalidate the HYP.

It took me many years of study and practice of the Hatha verses to gradually 'untranslate' the verses for myself, by looking at the Sanskrit terms, understanding the principles behind the Sanskrit terms and verifying the verses in my practice. I do experience the vayus, nadis, chakras, granthis and sushumna, and my students experience these phenomena too when I present them with the 'untranslated' wisdom. I believe the verses need to be studied in Sanskrit and practised to find the real Hatha Yoga.

I have translated the verses I use in this book myself, unless stated otherwise. I left the crucial terms untranslated; these are words that refer to experiences that don't have clear Western equivalents. The untranslated Sanskrit terms are explained in the text and also in the glossary at the end of the book. I translated the verses as literally as possible which sacrifices at some points the smooth flow of the language.

Chapter 3

PRANA

Before describing pranayama, we need to look in more detail at the principle of Prana, the force expanding in the process of pranayama. Prana is life, and wherever life is, there is Prana.

Prana is the most obvious phenomenon there is, but it is difficult for us to comprehend because we were brought up creating Western mind-patterns. Understanding is generally based on mind-patterns. The Sanskrit term is 'samskara', defined as 'latent impression, predisposition' in John Grimes' (1996) dictionary and defined and explored in the Yoga Sutras of Patanjali. Samskara is a framework within the mind, most of which is established in early childhood. Children do not question presented knowledge. Facts are given by parents, teachers and society, and these facts form the foundation for all further learning; they are usually not reviewed. An example of a common samskara in our society is 'it is important to be successful'. This belief might never be questioned throughout a person's whole life, remaining the driving force even when it causes unhappiness, relationship breakdown and ill health. Imagine a society based on the samskara 'it is important to develop spiritually in life' – lives would be lived very differently. Another example of a Western samskara is 'what cannot be seen does not exist'; when we are in doubt, we use the phrase 'I have to see it with my own eyes'. This is deeply ingrained in our understanding even though we know that our senses are limited. Animals can see different colours; bats can hear frequencies we cannot.

Prana cannot be seen, so holding the samskara 'I have to see it with my own eyes' causes us to disregard the entire concept. And yet we practise Yoga and pranayama. Not comprehending Prana, we modify the practice to fit an understandable pattern; we expand our lung capacity and call it pranayama. Prana has no space in a Western mental framework. The Yoga way of thinking is based on different samskaras and sees the phenomenon of Prana as an obvious expression of the cosmos.

Samskaras determine the way a culture perceives the universe

At this point, I would like to discuss the differences between the basic samskaras forming Western and Yoga cosmology and understandings of what the universe is and how it came to be. What this will show is that Western philosophical foundations have no space for a principle like Prana, and an incorrect interpretation of pranayama is bound to follow.

Western cosmology is based on the Judeo-Christian belief system, which has its roots in the Old Testament creation narratives. Chapter 2 of Genesis (the first book of Moses in the Old Testament) describes solid matter as having always been there, not created. God, an entity distinct from matter, forms the matter into manifestations that we experience as this universe, as a potter forms clay. Humans are distinct from other creations because they have a soul. The principle of change – transforming, growing, evolving – which is the principle of life, has no space in this mindset.

Humans, created by God, go through different stages of development, from embryo to child to adult. 'Which of these forms did God create?' was a serious question asked by medieval theologians. Today, humans are still seen as a set 'construction', which does not evolve or change. For this reason, it was difficult for Christians to accept Darwin's theory of evolution. The Christian samskara could not reconcile God and evolution. Did God create us or did we evolve? Today's medical science is still based on the premise of humans being a 'construction' and not a 'life process'. When we consult a doctor, we are offered surgery or drugs to repair the body's mechanisms; the inert healing process is seen as irrelevant.

In Yoga understanding, evolving, transforming, growing, changing is nature. Everything is alive, evolving, led by an inherent force, a divine force, Prana.

Prana cannot be seen, touched or thought, but it obviously *is*; otherwise, there is no life, evolution and growth. Evolution is a divine process; God is not a transcendent being outside the universe, but the force within it. Why does a leaf grow? Science can describe the chemical process of 'how the leaf grows', but not *why*. The Indian Yogis, not getting lost in the detail of 'how the leaf grows', saw the mysterious drive and movement within the universe: a principle that makes leaves grow and causes humans to mature, forests to cover the ground and galaxies to expand. This force also causes leaves to wilt, humans to age, forests to rot into humus and galaxies to be sucked into black holes.

I love the old English nursery rhyme below that expresses a simple wisdom, not much acknowledged in our scientific thinking:

Oats and beans and barley grow,
oats and beans and barley grow,
do you or I or anyone know
how oats and beans and barley grow?

(OLD ENGLISH NURSERY RHYME)

This is a simple and true statement showing the mystery behind all life, which we cannot explain. This mystery can be named or left unnamed; the Yogis call it Prana. This force creates a universe (srishti – the initial creation) as it expands, makes it evolve (sthiti – sustenance of creation), then retreats and causes decay (pralaya – decay, destruction, death). Western culture has seen the universe as solid matter, an unchangeable pot made by the potter, whereas for the Indian Yogis the universe is a process, permanent change and movement, which only *appears* to be in solid form. Rather, it is 'maya', a term that is described as 'the force which shows the unreal as real' (Grimes 1996).

The Sanskrit word 'maya' also means 'magic'. As a magician conjures a rabbit out of a hat even though the rabbit is not really in the hat, this apparent universe is not the ultimate reality. Matter consists of molecules, molecules consist of atoms, and atoms are just empty space in motion. This motion is Prana.

The great and the individual Prana, Maha Prana and vayu

Shakti or Prana is moving and evolving to create the appearance of the solid world. The Indians knew long before Einstein that matter is motion; matter is not fixed solidly, but is in permanent flux and flow. This is Maha Prana, the great Prana, which is the basis of all apparent existence. This Prana is 'the force which exists in all things, whether animate or inanimate' (Swami Satyananda Saraswati 1996a, p.363).

Maha Prana upholds the appearance of all objects whether animate or inanimate. What is an animate object? The root of the word is the Latin 'animus', which means 'psyche or spirit'. There are existences that have a spirit, such as humans, animals, plants, which we call animate. Those without an individual spirit, like rocks, stones and oceans, we call inanimate. However, they all have Maha Prana; all are a whirling process of electrons. Some of these pranic forms have spirit, an individual, conscious Self-awareness, which is bound into a form for a specific length of time we call life. This force that binds Spirit or Self into a form is individual Prana.

The Hatha Yogis work with individual Prana. Both a living body and a dead body maintain their form by Maha Prana being present in them. Without that force, the atoms would collapse. The difference between a living and a dead body is that the former contains a force holding consciousness within. Individual Prana is the force that binds consciousness or Shiva (Self, Atman, Purusha) to the body. Death occurs when that individualized Prana leaves and the link between the body and the consciousness breaks. The dead body matter is still a process of Maha Prana, which then modifies and transforms into humus.

The Hatha compositions refer to the movement of individual Prana with the term 'vayu' (wind). Vayu has five forms; there is a sixth form of individual Prana, kundalini, which I will define later.

At the beginning of a life the 'constant motion (vayu) commences as soon as we are conceived in our mother's womb' (Swami Niranjananda Saraswati 2002, p.580). It makes us evolve and grow, then it retreats and death occurs. 'Life is said to exist only so long as there is vayu in the body. Its departure is death' (HYP 2, 3). Individual life is the process of vayu binding consciousness, Self (Atman), into the body. It is the individual Prana that is relevant to exploring pranayama, and this is what I will be referring to from onwards.

Prana and Atman

Prana, also referred to as Shakti in Indian mythology, is only one element of the Divine, the element in constant movement creating the illusion of solidity. Behind the movement is an intent, an intelligence, consciousness, Shiva. Many names are given to that conscious core of everything: Shiva, Ishvara, Brahman and Krishna. The whole universe, Maha Prana, the Divine Shakti, is pervaded by consciousness, the Divine Brahman. Each individual being is conscious, and that individual consciousness does not differ from the universal consciousness. Individual consciousness is Atman, Purusha and, in most English translations, 'Self'. In an unenlightened state, the individual is not aware of being connected with the whole of the universe on the consciousness level. Enlightenment is the realization that Atman is Brahman.

Prana is not Atman, Purusha, Shiva or the Divine Consciousness. Prana is Shakti, life expanding and retreating, an ever-changing process. Purusha is unchanging; Prana causes creation and decay. Purusha is consciousness, the intelligence behind the pranic movement, that gives it a direction and intent. According to the Vedanta philosophy, Atman, Brahman, Purusha, Self or even 'the Lord' is the only lasting reality and out of this reality arises Prana.

Prana is the life force that allows the Self or consciousness to stay linked to the bodily system and experience life.

> When the body and the mind grow weak, the Self gathers in all the powers of life [vayus] and descends with them into the heart. As prana leaves the eye, it ceases to see…he [the body] no longer hears; he no longer speaks, or tastes, or smells or thinks or knows. By the light of the heart the Self leaves the body by one of its gates; and when he leaves, prana follows, and with it all the vital powers of the body. (Easwaran 1988, Brihadaranyaka Upanishad IV, 4.2)

As long as vayu moves in the eye, the Self experiences seeing; as long as vayu moves in the ear, the Self experiences hearing. Death breaks the link between Self and body; the vayu retreats.

Prana and breath

Individual Prana comes in six forms. Of the five vayus, four move in rhythm with the breath. They are apana, samana, prana and udana (see the section 'Vayu (wind)' below). The fifth vayu, vyana is an expanding pranic force independent of the breathing rhythm; it moves whenever the pranic body is purifying and takes up the cleared space – just as the sun shines into all the spaces where shade is removed. The sixth individual Prana is the dormant kundalini that becomes awake when the physical breath stops.

Prana is not breath, and only four of the six forms are related to the breath by sharing the same rhythm.

Prana is an element that gives life, and death occurs by its absence. English versions of Yoga verses translate the term 'Prana' with 'breath', but Prana is not breath, even though the two phenomena are linked. Breath is the bodily rhythm that causes the movement of four vayus as well as the movement of respiration, air moving in and out of the lungs.

From here on, I will use the term 'breath' to refer to the bodily rhythm. The process of airflow I will call 'respiration'. The process of the subtle shift of pranic fields, which happens in the same rhythm as respiration, I will call 'vayu movement' or pranayama.

Let me share the following analogy I use when teaching pranayama. An orchestra is playing along to a given beat – the waving of the arms of a conductor, the breath. Initiated by the wave of the conductor's arms, the violins play – the respiration. Independent from the violins – but in harmony with them, and also following the rhythm of the conductor's arms – is the playing of the clarinets: different players, different instruments, different notes – the vayu. The clarinets and the violins are linked together by the conductor's arm movements; in the same way, the breath links the respiration and the vayu together and keeps them in harmony with each other, but they are substantially different. And there are even more instruments playing in the orchestra: a harp, for example. In his commentary on the Yoga Sutras, Iyengar explains that awareness is moving from the inner core through all the koshas, the five sheaths of the human body, in the rhythm of the breath. Awareness moves during the inhalation from the most internal kosha to the outer physical sheath and returns to the deepest layers with the exhalation

(Iyengar 1991). Respiration is the movement that the breath initiates in the annamaya kosha, the physical body. Vayu is the movement breath initiates in pranamaya kosha, the pranic body, and the shift of awareness is the movement breath initiates throughout all layers.

Respiration is one function of that 'breath', a function the Yogis were not concerned with. No Yoga composition gives descriptions of respiration; there are no words to describe the lungs, diaphragm, oxygen, air moving through the nostrils. Looking in a dictionary for a Sanskrit term for the English word 'nostril', we find quite a few words. None of these words are used in any Hatha composition in the context of pranayama. The Hatha compositions are nevertheless full of words describing the vayu movement. The Hatha Yogis did not know the science of respiration and were not interested in it. Breath for them was the experience of a subtle shift of Prana from the mid-abdomen outwards and back.

At the same time as air is drawn into the lungs (inhalation), the vayu expands out from manipura, and at the same time as air is released from the lungs (exhalation), the vayu reverts to manipura. We are *not* taking Prana from the atmosphere with an inhalation. Prana is within. We are *not* recharging our body with Prana. We are *not* breathing because we run out of Prana.

Nadi

Vayu moves in the subtle body, pranamaya kosha, and uses pathways called nadis (pulses, arteries, tubes; in the Hatha context: prana conductor). In Chinese medicine, the equivalent of nadis are called meridians, channels for Chi, which is very much the same as Prana. There are no detectable channels in the physical body. We talk about channels for energy when referring to meridians, but Prana is not really energy, and it is therefore better to speak of Prana conductors (conductor in the sense of a substance that allows electricity to flow through). When the Hatha teachings first came to the West, we looked for nadis in the human anatomy. We looked for conductors, which keep this whole bodily system going, keeps it connected and functioning, and we found nerves. Nerves are realities in the anatomical body, annamaya kosha, and detectable with microscopes. Nerves conduct impulses from the brain to all body parts instructing movement, perception and the sensation of pain. Nadis are not detectable with a microscope; they are realities of the pranic body, pranamaya kosha. Nadis do not carry impulses through the body, but are pathways for vayu, the subtler element maintaining the connection of consciousness with the living organism. We still find Yoga books today, some even written by Indians, speaking about the pranic force flowing through the nerves.

> The term nadi should be properly understood. Nerves and nadis are two different things. Nerves relate to the physical body, whereas nadis relate to the pranic. (Swami Niranjananda Saraswati 2002, pp.58-59)

Life force does not move arbitrarily, but follows a pattern, the nadis. The HYP claims the existence of 72,000 patterns, nadis (HYP 1, 39; 3, 123; 4, 18); other texts such as the Siva Samitha speak of 350,000 (2, 13). Unlike Chinese culture, which devised detailed charts of the meridians, Indian culture did not show much interest in such detail. The main purpose of the Indian Yoga system is spiritual awakening, and the interest centred therefore mainly on one nadi, the middle one, the most gracious one – sushumna. An unblocked flow of life force in sushumna leads to spiritual awakening. None of the Indian compositions, as far as we know, give a complete description of the whole nadi system. There are nevertheless references to the origin point of all nadis, which sits in manipura chakra: 'All 72000 nadis originate from kanda, which is like a bird's egg' (Feuerstein 2001, p.401, quoting the Goraksha Paddhati).

Just as life is hatched from a bird's egg, so does life arise from the origin of all nadis. Kanda (piece) is not a chakra, but is found in the region of a chakra. This region is the centre point of all life evolving: 'Where kanda is strung on sushumna, like a jewel on a thread, that region is called manipoora chakra' (Feuerstein 2001, p.401, quoting the Goraksha Paddhati).

Most Hatha Yoga compositions name only three nadis. The Shiva Samitha, the Shiva Swarodaya and others describe and locate 14, which are situated in similar places as the main meridians in the Chinese system. The three nadis important to the Hatha tradition are ida (the word has no meaning in Sanskrit other than the name of this nadi), pingala (brown) and sushumna (gracious). Ida is positioned on the left side in the pranic body and connects to all nadis on the left. Pingala is positioned on the right and connects to all nadis on the right. Those two nadis merge in ajna chakra, the third eye, and make up the **outer pranic body**.

A teaching that most Yoga teachers have received is that ida, together with the associated nadis on the left side, is connected to the right side of the brain and is therefore responsible for the intuitive, female, moon side of us. Pingala, along with the associated nadis on the right, is connected to the left side of the brain and is therefore responsible for the intellectual, male, sun side of us. We were taught this because our teachers tried to match the pranic process with anatomy. The nerves on the left side of the spinal cord are connected to the right side of the brain and vice versa. The pranic process does not take place in the physical body, and no Hatha composition suggests a crossover. All nadis of the left and all nadis on the right merge in ajna chakra, the third eye, not in the brain. Between ajna and saharsrara, the opening of the pranic body at the crown of the head, is only one nadi, sushumna; there is no right or left side.

Sushumna is of the highest significance. Vayu moves in the rhythm of the breath in ida and pingala and their connected nadis. When the vayus fully reverse (see the section 'Vayu (wind)' below) the collision of the pranic fields releases power, which opens the entrance of sushumna at the base chakra, muladhara. Kundalini (see the section 'What is kundalini?' in Chapter 4), a dormant high frequency of Prana, awakens and starts rising up sushumna, **the inner pranic body**. The gradual movement of the kundalini force up sushumna awakens all the main chakras and progresses the practitioner on the path of human evolution with the goal of 'enlightenment'.

Vayu (wind)

Not many students visiting Yoga classes in the West report being taught vayus, but without the understanding and experience of vayu, authentic pranayama cannot take place. Swami Satyananda Saraswati, the founder of the Bihar School of Yoga and publisher of many books on Yoga, bases his understanding on the pranic body. He was one of only a few Yoga masters in more modern times who taught the vayu in detail, and so did his students. One book describes

> the pranic body, which is comprised of the individual prana and the network of nadis which carry this prana; it is divided into five main areas or sub-pranas. These are collectively known as the pancha (five) pranas: prana, apana, samana, udana and vyana. (Swami Niranjananda Saraswati 2002, p.62)

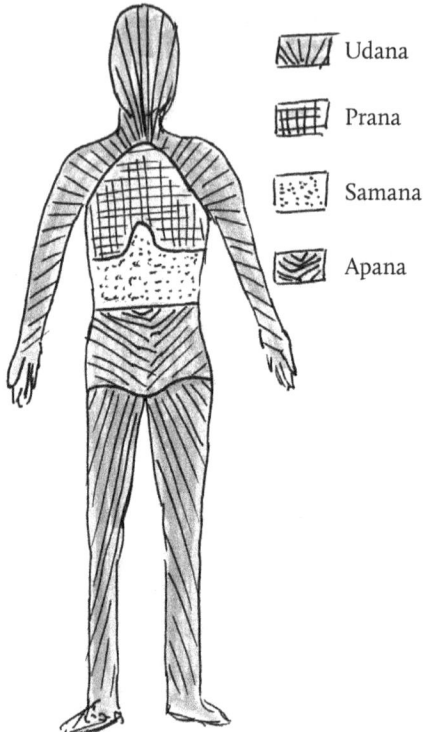

Figure 3.1 *The pranic body*

Detailed descriptions of the vayus are already found in one of the earliest works of the Hatha tradition, the Goraksha Paddhati. The location of the vayus has not changed since:

> Prana, apana, samana, udana as well as vyana are the principal winds... Prana dwells at the heart, apana is always in the region of the anus, samana is the location of the navel, udana is in the middle of the throat... vyana pervades the whole body. These are the 5 principal winds. (Feuerstein 2001, p. 404)

The five main vayus

The vayus move in the pranic body. Vayu is not made of Prana; it is a movement in Prana. In the same way, wind is not made of air, but it moves through air.

In order to describe the direction of the movement, words are needed to point to the regions of the Prana flow. Swami Satyananda Saraswati uses physical terms to describe the process in the pranic body, which I will use here as well, in the absence of other vocabulary. When I speak about the chest, I do not mean the ribcage with the lungs, but the region above manipura, and when I speak about the pelvis, I do not mean the lower body organs, but the region below manipura.

We can use physical terms in the way we use a map for finding a location. The dots and lines on the map are not the place itself, just a way to find it. Once 'arrived' in the location, one experiences the area directly and the map can be discarded. In the same way, we can drop the physical terms when we have arrived at the pranic experience. I instruct my students to 'let the breath expand outward from the mid-abdomen and then reverse back', and I am not referring to respiration or guts. When my students have gained the direct experience, then I can change the instruction to 'let vayu expand from kanda and reverse back'.

Prana (when referring to the sub-vayu, it is usually written with a small 'p' to distinguish it from Prana as a whole) is the wave moving from kanda upwards into the chest region. The expansion of prana outwards into the chest region occurs at the same time as the inhalation and should not to be mistaken for thoracic breathing. Thoracic breathing is a function of the respiratory system, an emergency mechanism, kicking in when the brain registers low levels of oxygen. The intercostal muscles, the small muscles sitting between the ribs, contract and widen the ribcage to allow a higher airflow into the lungs. The movement of prana in the chest region is not widening the ribcage. It is not prana expansion when the chest rises while breathing. The inhalation happening simultaneously with the prana expansion remains purely diaphragmatic. Prana vayu is of a much more subtle nature than air.

Apana is the wave moving from kanda into the pelvic region. Apana is a good starting point when learning to experience the vayus, because no respiration takes place below the navel. A sensation of a movement and aliveness down into the pelvis and back cannot so easily be mistaken for respiration. Simultaneous with inhalation, in the same rhythm as the breath, apana moves downs into the pelvis and returns into the navel centre as the exhalation happens.

One of my Yoga teacher colleagues told me that her teacher taught breathing into the pelvis and legs. One of her students questioned the practice as no respiration is taking place in the legs and pelvis. The teacher explained the practice with the term 'internal respiration', which is the distribution of oxygen in the blood system throughout the whole body after the gas exchange in the lungs. This answer seemed to satisfy everyone, but it is not correct. Vayu moves Prana in the pranic body, whereas internal respiration moves oxygen through the physical body. The questioning student felt the movement but needed an anatomical explanation. Internal respiration cannot be felt and it does not happen in the rhythm of the breath, or in any rhythm at all. Apana can be felt in the rhythm of the breath. The apana reverse is of specific importance. Apana shifts back up as prana moves down; those two vayus meet in the middle when the reverse is complete.

> Rising the apana upward and bringing the prana down from the throat, the yogi becomes free from old age as if 16 years of age. (HYP 2, 47)

Samana is the vayu moving sidewards from manipura and back, in the area below the diaphragm. Samana can be mistaken for respiration as the abdominal area moves outwards during inhalation. The diaphragm, which is shaped like a dome, contracts upwards and flattens downwards during inhalation to create a vacuum in the lungs for air to draw in. The down-moving diaphragm compresses the abdominal organs and moves the abdominal wall outwards. This outwards movement is not samana. Samana expands life force through the pranic body, not the physical body. Samana is, like prana and apana, a much more subtle substance than air. The vayu movement is more tangible and more complete when the airflow is decreased to nearly nothing and the abdominal wall is hardly moving. It takes practice to experience the difference between abdominal breath and samana; it helps to widen the nostrils to reduce airflow and keep the chin low, applying Jalandhara bandha.

I have attended 'pranayama' days where participants were asked to place their hands on the abdomen, then on the sides and on the lower back to feel the movement. This is a useful practice to develop a more reliable diaphragmatic breath, which is a prerequisite of pranayama, but it is not pranayama. Movement you feel with the hands on the physical body is not samana.

Udana has been experienced and taught by Swami Satyananda Saraswati as the shifting force from manipura into head and arms and legs (see Swami Niranjanananda Saraswati 2002, p.60). No one can mistake udana as respiration, unless you refer to internal respiration; it moves into the extremities in the rhythm of the breath. It is nevertheless a difficult vayu to connect to; the breathing rhythm needs to slow down considerably to be able to follow the complete movement of the vayu outwards to feet, hands and head, and then back. To experience udana, one needs to have reduced airflow and be able to remain in a pause after the vayu reverse, kumbhaka. Udana reaches further than the other vayus, and the pranic body needs a high level of purification to experience udana. A more purified pranic body allows the practitioner to perceive layers deeper than the anatomical. Being in touch with udana is therefore a spiritual advance, as seen in the Prashna Upanishad:

> Udana, the fifth force, leads the selfless up the ladder of evolution, and the selfish down. (Easwaran 1988, Prashna Upanishad, Question II, 7)

Vayu is subtle but very powerful; it can be felt but cannot be seen or detected with a microscope. Insight into the vayu movement can only be gained through introspection and determined practice of Hatha Yoga, the science of experience and exploration of the pranic body. It is not that difficult to feel the vayu; most of my students get a sense of vayu pretty quickly when instructed to drop the usual mind framework (samskara).

We all feel the vayu movement, but do not reflect on it. We would otherwise not refer to diaphragmatic breath as 'abdominal breath'. Respiration does not occur in the abdomen; the abdominal wall will move outwards during inhalation as the diaphragm flattens downwards, not because the belly fills with air. We cannot feel the diaphragm moving; if we did, then it would be felt as a downward pressure on our guts, but not as an expansion from the mid-abdomen. I have heard many people who lack anatomical knowledge referring to diaphragmatic breath as 'breathing air into the belly'. Why? Because we feel the belly as the centre of breath and it is expanding during the inhalation.

When I am running workshops for Yoga teachers on pranayama, some participants often raise the objection that we cannot possibly teach subtle processes like vayu to beginners. One certainly can, and I do. I instruct beginners straight away to pay attention to the movement from the mid-abdomen and tell them that 'breath' in Yoga is different from respiration. It is actually easier to teach vayu to beginners than to students who have had lots of training with 'respiration pranayama', because beginners come without preconceptions of what Yoga is, whereas advanced students struggle to let go of their mind-patterns (samskaras).

A commonly used analogy for the vayu is that of water flowing through pipes. This analogy is quite mechanistic and not very helpful. The pranic process is much more subtle: the vayus move through Prana like a wave that moves through the water. Watching ripples or waves in the sea, we see waves moving towards us, but the water does not; otherwise, any object floating on the sea would be carried to the shore immediately. The waves move through the water; the waves are not water, but can only move where there is water. The vayus do not shift Prana through the pranic body, from one place to the other; they move through Prana and can only move where there is Prana. Practising the vayu movement can become forced and ineffective when we try to actively shift the life force into depleted areas. Vayu does not have material quality; it is just a subtle flicker through the pranic body.

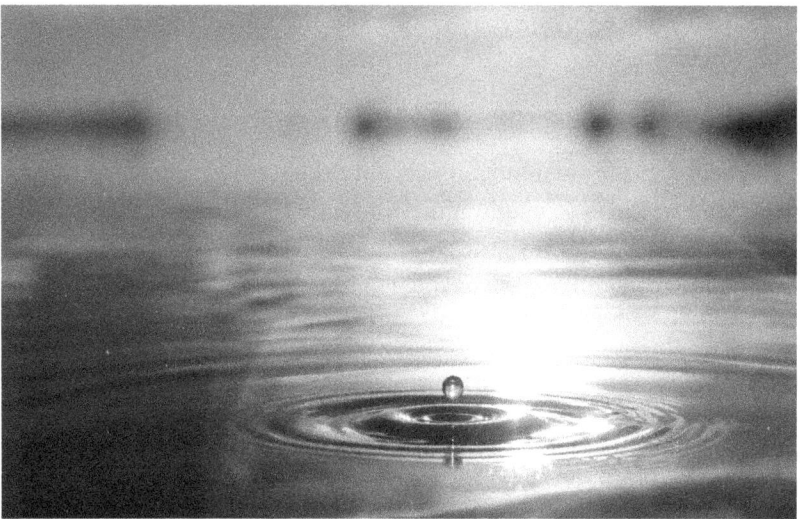

Figure 3.2 *Waves moving through the water*

One might ask why the Yogis used four different names to describe a movement in four different directions instead of saying vayu moves up, down, sidewards and into the extremities. There is a reason. Vayus, like waves, differ from each other. Each wave has its own specific frequency – the number of risings and falls per minute – and amplitude – the height of the wave. In the same way, vayus differ. Apana will have a different 'frequency and amplitude' from prana, samana and udana. The difference cannot be measured, but it can be felt, and it is difficult to find words to match the sense of each individual vayu. Some people express the difference in colours; I personally see apana in a more yellow shade, samana in orange, prana in light blue and udana in a very light green. One can link the differences to the qualities of the elements: apana feels earthy, samana fiery, prana watery and udana airy.

These are the four vayus: prana, apana, samana and udana, the waves moving through the pranic body in the rhythm of the breath. There is also a fifth.

Vyana has a different nature – a sense of flickering aliveness in all the areas that have received purification by the other four vayus. Vyana is independent of breath, as Prana itself is; it is a still movement in a stationary form, like electrons racing around the nucleus of an atom which itself stands still. Everyone feels it, and Yoga practitioners usually refer to the sensation with the words 'nice', 'beautiful' or 'relaxed', without reflecting on the nature of the sensation. By practising Yoga with focus on the vayu movement, we can feel a change within. Some people say they feel their body parts are longer, higher, heavier, lighter. None of this is the case: when considering the physical body, it is the same as before; the difference is the invisible aliveness that expands into the cleared areas, a more active vyana.

Some traditions, like the Shiva Samhita, distinguish ten vayus, five major and five minor. The five major are as described above, the minor ones are naga (belching), kurma (opening the eyes), krkara (hunger and thirst), devadatta (yawning) and dhanajnayah (hiccup). How those functions are related to the movement of the first five vayus is not explained and not obvious.

Refrain

Pranayama is not respiration, but the expansion of Prana. Pranayama is a process not in the physical body but in the pranic body. Prana is not air or breath, but life that enters each embryo and settles in the navel centre; death occurs when Prana, life, leaves.

Pranayama, the expansion of Prana, is a threefold process: (1) the expanding of Prana from its origin in the navel centre outwards; (2) the reversing of Prana back to the navel centre; and (3) the containing of Prana in the navel centre. The threefold process is called vayu, and it happens in the rhythm of the breath, but it is not breath, and it moves in the opposite direction to respiration. Vayu does not move through air tubes but through nadis. The nadis are full of impurities, and pranayama is the purification process. Once the nadis are purified, the vayu stops moving and breath ceases. Prana then remains for prolonged periods in the navel centre where it creates heat, which awakens a dormant pranic force sitting in the base chakra, kundalini. Kundalini rises in the innermost, spiritual nadi, sushumna; when it reaches the top, sahasrara, an enlightened state occurs.

The origin of vayu, manipura

All our active life force resides in **manipura chakra** (the city of jewels, the bright shining place, the third chakra, located in the mid-abdomen), the storehouse of Prana. The fine network of prana conductors, the nadis, all have their origin in the same area. When they refer to the storehouse of Prana, the Hatha Yogis call it **manipura**. In the context of the origin point of the nadis, the term **kanda** (trunk, stem, bulb, the place from where growth outwards comes from) is used. When the pranic movement is less disturbed, heat and power are felt in the same area, then the Hatha Yogis referred to the experience of heat in the mid-abdomen with the term **agni** (fire). Manipura, kanda and agni are all experiences linked to the same location. This place is an experience and not a tangible reality, and all factual knowledge about it is useless, if not misleading.

Some years ago, I participated in a seven-day course on chakras – one chakra per day. We looked at the symbolism of each chakra, the Sanskrit mantras, the associated elements and animals. At the end of the course, I did not feel any closer to a direct understanding of chakras than before, and I was under the impression that there was nothing more I could do to grasp the phenomenon of chakra. The course supplied us with knowledge of the chakras, not the direct experience. To gain direct understanding, we need to sit and look, apply practices that can unblock the areas and bring us into better connection, and not think or know. Thinking about a chakra gives us the expectation of a tangible reality in a three-dimensional space; we don't find it and so we conclude that we cannot feel chakras. Everyone can feel chakras, but as a subtle non-material and non-locatable sensation. The pranic body is not situated in the third dimension, but in deeper ones, which are not accessible by our imagination and thought, but by direct perception.

When a human is conceived, two cells merge and multiply. That organism is growing in the mother's body and, at the beginning, it is part of the mother's body. At some point, it becomes an own life form; there is speculation about when this form becomes an individual being. Swami Satyananda Saraswati's school assumes it is the moment of conception: 'constant motion (vayu) commences as soon as we are conceived in our mother's womb' (Swami Niranjananda Saraswati 2002, p.580).

Tibetan Buddhism, however, dates the beginning of the individual life of the embryo on day 49, seven weeks; on this day it is believed that the soul enters the organism.

Western science knows that the umbilical cord starts to form by the third week after conception, and it is completed to connect the foetus with the placenta at seven weeks, the same time the Buddhists assume that the soul enters.

The navel centre, as the name suggests, is located just behind the navel. The navel is the scar left from the umbilical cord. I feel it is therefore feasible to believe that Prana enters the embryo through the mother's body via the umbilical cord as soon as it is connected. The timing agrees with Buddhist wisdom and also with anthropologist Rudolf Steiner. According to Steiner, a major change occurs at the seventh the week of pregnancy: 'in the first period after conception, only the causal body is active in the human germ; around the seventh week the etheric body begins its descent' (Free Man Creator 2024). The descent of the etheric body is, according to Steiner, when the little organism becomes an individual, its own life, the soul being connected to the bodily form by Prana.

I believe that life enters the little organism through the umbilical cord, which is by then one centimetre long. The point of entrance is later marked by the navel. Prana forms the place the Yogis describe as manipura, kanda, agni, and the constant movement of the vayu commences.

Practical: connect to the movement of the vayus
Do not practise all directions at the same time, but just one at a time. Revisit the practice daily for a few minutes and move on to the next vayu when you feel confident.

Get a sense of the vayus
Give yourself some time and choose a quiet place. Apply a seated posture that you can maintain undisturbed for a few minutes. Close your eyes and withdraw your senses from the outside; be aware of the inner space. When you witness your thought processes becoming calmer, bring your focus to the respiration, air flowing from the outside through the nostrils into the lungs and then from the lungs through the nostrils back to the atmosphere. Continue for a while, then lead the centre of your awareness to the mid-abdomen. Allow a few extended exhalations to drop your focus into the mid-abdomen, to move your centredness from the head into the navel centre. Feel an expansion outwards at the time of the inhalation and a reverse back to the mid-abdomen at the time of the exhalation, the vayu. Try to focus on this movement, which is subtler than respiration; no longer allow respiration be part of your inner 'seeing'. If your focus becomes sharp, you might get confused and no longer know which move is inhalation and which exhalation. That is a good sign: you are really connecting to vayu. Apply a soft ujjayi; the throaty sound is very useful for establishing a better focus on the vayu movement. Drop ujjayi when your focus is steady and replace it with a soft 'air-free' and sound-free movement. Widen the nostrils, which will reduce the airflow and as such intensify the vayu.

> **Note:** The technique of widening the nostrils has often been taught to help the pranayama experience. I remember having been told that widening the nostrils would open them for higher air and Prana intake. I believe this argument to be flawed: first, Prana is within and is not taken from the atmosphere; second, airflow is reduced when widening the nostrils. Narrowing the nostrils, as we do when blowing our nose, increases the air volume and speed. Widening the nostrils is a wonderful technique to reduce airflow and thus intensify the perception of vayu. I am sure those teachers

who taught this technique felt the effect of pranic increase; they just interpreted it differently.

Carry on and become absorbed.

Now change back to respiration; feel the air from outside flowing through the nostrils into the lungs, then back out of the nostrils into the atmosphere. You should feel a very different 'breath'. The locations of the two processes are different: respiration in the head, chest and outside; vayu in the abdominal region. Respiration is an exchange between the inside and outside; vayu is only inside. Respiration feels extraverted, the vayu introverted. Respiration is a gross process working with the element air; vayu is a subtle, non-physical experience.

Apana vayu
When you are confident that you can connect to the vayu, differentiate the practice by focusing on individual vayus one by one. Start with apana (this is the easiest). Sit still in a comfortable posture, settle your awareness in the navel centre, and watch the vayu. When your focus is steady, concentrate solely on the downwards movement. I do find it useful at this point to show students a skeleton and ask them to visualize the 'bowl of bones' – the pelvis – even though the vayu does not move in the physical body. Feel apana expanding down and filling the whole pelvic bowl, then imagine reaching down with two invisible hands into the pelvic bowl to gather up the subtle substance and bring it back to the mid-abdomen. Apana moves like a wind and carries life like wind carries a scent which fills the lower pranic body. At first this might just be a visualization, but the visualization will soon be replaced by an actual perception of the process. At this point, drop the image of the bowl of bones.

> **Note:** The Hatha instructions stress the importance of the reversing of the apana and prana for the two fields to meet (see HYP 2, 47). Not only can habitual breathing prevent the expansion of vayu, but also the reverse can be blocked by inattentiveness.

Use the image of the invisible hands again, but this time do not gather up apana to reverse it, but imagine turning your hands around, palms down. The vayu, the wind moving back to the navel centre, leaving life behind. See whether you can feel the reverse lacking an aliveness – the return feels empty. One of my students used the word 'stale' to describe the sensation of the 'empty' apana reverse, and she referred to the complete apana reversing with the words 'like flowing fresh spring water'.

Samana vayu
Samana does not cause the physical movement of the abdomen and the sides; respiration does this simultaneously to samana movement. Widen the nostrils to reduce the airflow, moving the chin towards the throat without dropping the head, and apply kechari mudra (tip of the tongue towards the back of the mouth). You will feel the sense of a much subtler and slower expansion, which can carry on when the abdominal movement, caused by diaphragmatic breath, has stopped. Let the reverse flow like a stream back to the origin of all the nadis.

Prana vayu
Prana vayu can be mistaken for thoracic breathing. When focusing on an upwards movement during the inhalation, the tendency is to breathe air into the chest. Make sure you maintain diaphragmatic respiration. Do not aim for an expanding of the ribcage with air, but a sensation of a subtle shining, a livening; you will have a feeling of inward awareness. The subtle experience upwards takes place in a plane beneath the physical, not in annamaya, but in pranamaya kosha. Keep the nostrils widened, move the centre of your awareness into the mid-abdomen and witness the movement from there. As prana shifts upwards, refrain from 'going along' with it. Imagine that your inner witness is like a source of light: the light shines upwards, but you keep the source of light where it is. Feel the reverse of prana as a stream downwards; let it flow. Experiencing prana requires a straight posture; any misalignment of the pelvis creates barriers between chest and abdomen. Tilt the pelvis forward and backwards a few times; play with the posture to find the right position where the reverse is least disturbed.

Upana vayu

Upana, the vayu that moves in the limbs and head, begins like the other vayus in the navel centre. When the apana, samana and prana movement become less restricted through practice, when the breath has slowed and airflow reduced, then the movement of the vayu can expand further. Blockages in the area of the hips, shoulders and neck can prevent this expansion (remember that we work with the pranic body and not with the physical body, so do not visualize anatomical body parts). It is therefore useful to begin the udana practice with asana that purify the pranic areas in the region of hips, shoulders and neck.

After your asana practice, focus on the vayu movement and apply udana first standing in tadasana. Start in manipura and let the expansion travel to the legs, then the arms and head. Maintain an upright posture – do not sag during the reverse. Focus on the reverse right back to the navel centre and gradually establish a pause after arriving – kumbhaka. You will know whether you need to free more in hips, shoulders and neck: it is when udana still feels restricted. With focused practice of udana, the physicality seems to disappear: stand with closed eyes and allow yourself to experience just being a wave of expanding outwards and back.

The next step is the combination of all four of those vayus and then the application of the complete vayu practice in asana. When you become able to add the refinement of the vayu movement to asana, your Yoga practice will transform. Yoga is no more stretching muscles: more and more, you will discover that you can access your pranic body, your sensations body, and you will be able to change it in a much more effective way.

Vyana vayu

> **Note:** Vyana is a beautiful experience for beginners and experienced practitioners alike. We all experience vyana; it is what makes us love Yoga. Vyana is what causes the first realizations for newcomers that Yoga differs from stretching. We know the sensation of vyana and usually call it a beautiful feeling, nothing more. We do not believe the sensation of vyana to be an indisputable

reality because there is no evidence of it in our anatomical body. Our physical body does not change when vyana expands, but we feel transformed. Vyana is not linked to the rhythm of the breath. Vyana is that form of Prana which expands on its own into all places that have been opened for it.

While focusing on the vayu movement, practise asana, preferably in the supine position, on the right side only. Hold each posture for up to a minute. You can use postures like those shown below.

Extend the right straight leg up to the ceiling, if you cannot reach use a belt (Figure 3.3), then lower it to the right side (Figure 3.4).

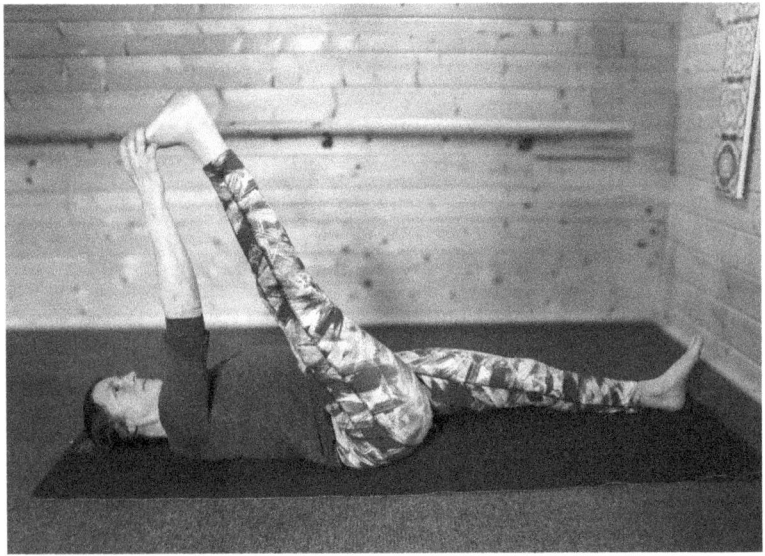

Figure 3.3 *Ardha urdhva mukha paschimottanasana*

Bend the knee and place the foot on the left knee, right arm out to the side, and drop the bended knee to the left towards the floor (Figure 3.5).

Bring the right knee further to the right, hold on to the right ankle with both hands, lift the head and lead the foot towards your head (Figure 3.6).

For the next posture, lift the right knee back to the chest, lift the lower leg up to the ceiling, bend and lower the knee towards the armpit (Figure 3.7).

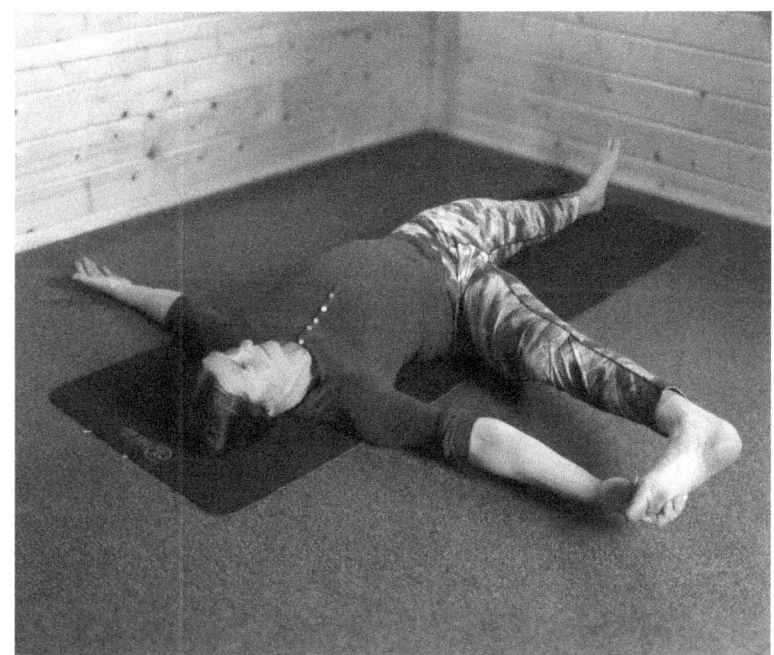

Figure 3.4 *Supta trikonasana*

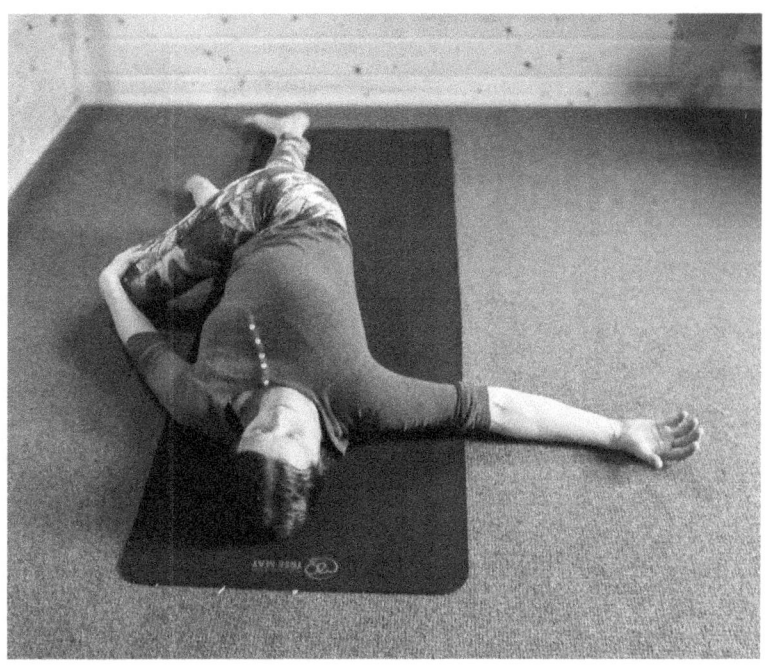

Figure 3.5 *Jathara parivrtti*

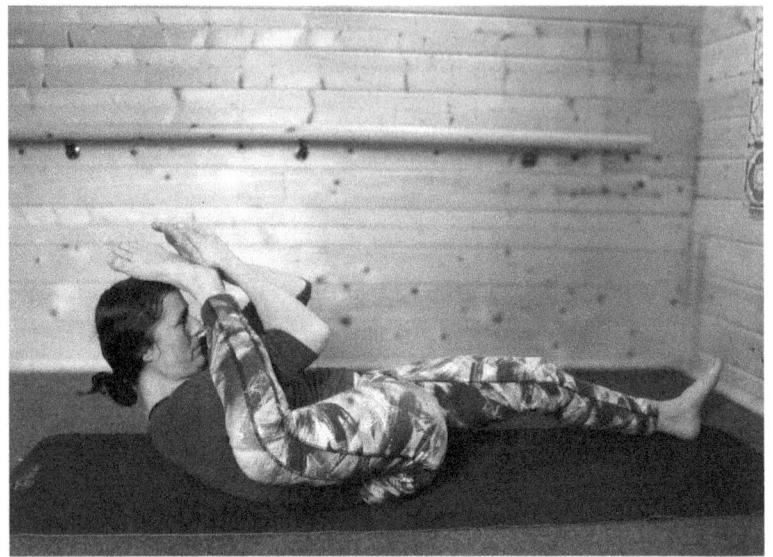

Figure 3.6 *Ardha yoganidrasana*

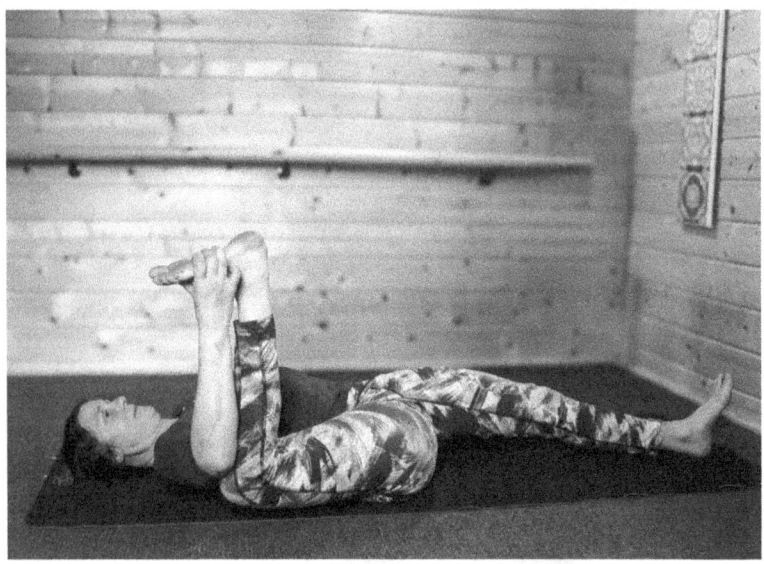

Figure 3.7 *Supta ashwa sanchalanasana*

You can use the above suggestion or any other asana sequence as long as you work on one side only.

Now lie in savasana and observe the right side of the body. A sensation of aliveness is seeping into the whole right side; the left side remains dull. The asana started a purification process of the nadis and the vayu of vyana can now enter the opened spaces. Take this experience as a real fact that you have discovered by the 'science of inner exploration', the science the Hatha Yogis applied to gain their knowledge.

Now apply the same sequence on the left side to even the vyana expansion throughout the whole system.

Refrain

Pranayama is not respiration, but the expansion of Prana. Pranayama is a process not in the physical body but in the pranic body. Prana is not air or breath, but life that enters each embryo and settles in the navel centre; death occurs when Prana, life, leaves.

Pranayama, the expansion of Prana, is a threefold process: (1) the expanding of Prana from its origin in the navel centre outwards; (2) the reversing of Prana back to the navel centre; and (3) the containing of Prana in the navel centre. The threefold process is called vayu, and it happens in the rhythm of the breath, but it is not breath, and it moves in the opposite direction to respiration. Vayu does not move through air tubes but through nadis. The nadis are full of impurities, and pranayama is the purification process. Once the nadis are purified, the vayu stops moving and breath ceases. Prana then remains for prolonged periods in the navel centre where it creates heat, which awakens a dormant pranic force sitting in the base chakra, kundalini. Kundalini rises in the innermost, spiritual nadi, sushumna; when it reaches the top, sahasrara, an enlightened state occurs.

Chapter 4

PRANAYAMA

So far, we have seen that pranayama, the expansion of life force, is a movement in the subtle body. This yogic wisdom has not survived in modern Western Yoga culture. A recent internet article on the site Femina states:

> Prana is the Sanskrit word for 'breath' and Yama means 'control'. As the name suggests, pranayama is the practice of controlling your breathing pattern in order to improve your physical and mental well-being. It involves inhaling, exhaling and holding your breath for a variety of different time intervals to remove carbon dioxide from your body and improve the flow of oxygen to the brain cells. This results in enhanced memory, focus and other cognitive abilities. (Ailani 2022)

I believe this definition loses sight of the original meaning of pranayama in the ancient Yoga tradition; unfortunately, this understanding of pranayama is the modern norm.

How pranayama is often taught in modern Yoga

The previous quotation expresses a common Western misunderstanding of pranayama. 'Prana' is not the Sanskrit word for 'breath'; Prana is the life within us. Pranayama is not concerned with controlling breathing patterns; pranayama is the expansion of the aliveness within us. Pranayama is not practised for physical and mental wellbeing but is a means to find an enlightened state and inner freedom. Pranayama is not inhaling, exhaling and holding the breath, but expanding the life force outwards and reversing back, and the third stage is not holding, but the transfer of the pranic force into a deeper, spiritual dimension, sushumna. Pranayama is not a practice to remove carbon dioxide and introduce oxygen; it actually aims for the cessation of breath. Enhancing memory, focus and cognitive abilities is not the aim of pranayama; pranayama is a spiritual practice which leads to a still mind, a state without any cognitive abilities.

Everyone is entitled to teach and promote breathing practices as they are described in the previously mentioned article, but they should not be called pranayama and linked to Yoga!

Understanding pranayama is not easy for us. The concept of Prana is difficult to comprehend for a Western mind, and vayu movement occurs in the same rhythm as respiration. Therefore, pranayama has been linked with respiration since the very first introduction of Hatha Yoga into the West.

Earlier, we looked at one of the first Western Yoga authors, André Van Lysebeth, who began his 1982 book, *Yoga*, with a chapter on breath. He did not use the word 'pranayama', which was the title of another book written by him ten years earlier in 1972. In the course of these ten years, he became a popular Yoga teacher and tried to adjust the discipline for a Western palate, as the subtitle indicates: *Yoga: für Menschen von heute* (Yoga for people of today's world). He instructed a practice that he called 'Die vollstandige Yogi-Atmung' (the complete Yoga-breath). This complete breath is the combination of all three respiratory capacities: the diaphragmatic breath, the thoracic breath and the clavicular breath. The complete breath is aiming for maximum air intake: 'Nun ist Ihre Lunge maximal mit Luft angefullt' [now your lungs are filled with the maximum amount of air] (Van Lysebeth 1982, p.47).

This three-part breath has been practised ever since, as other teachers adopted the practice, including Indian teachers such as Swami Niranjananda Saraswati, a student of Swami Satyananda Saraswati. He originally published his book *Prana Pranayama Prana Vidya* in 1994, 12 years after the appearance of Van Lysebeth's *Yoga*, and would have studied and applied Van Lysebeth's teaching.

> Yogic breathing commences inhalation with the diaphragm moving down to its maximum extent. This is followed by full thoracic then clavicular inhalation. The exhalation is the exact reverse of this, with a combination of diaphragmatic and thoracic compression of the lungs to complete the expulsion of the air. The lungs are stretched to maximum

capacity on both inhalation and exhalation. (Swami Niranjananda Saraswati 2002, p.133)

It is perfectly in order to practise and teach this breath, but I believe this is not Yoga and, more to the point, not pranayama. As respiration and pranayama share the same rhythm, the breath, there is inhalation and exhalation alongside pranayama. In pranayama practice, we do not manipulate respiration – in fact, we pay very little attention to it; rather, we are focusing on the vayu movement and purification of the nadis.

I suspect that Van Lysebeth must have developed this practice in the ten years between the two mentioned books: his first book, *Pranayama*, does not include the three-part breath.

As a Yoga learner, I have visited countless classes, Yoga days, courses and workshops. I have been given all sorts of information and instruction concerning pranayama, but most of all the instruction of the so-called 'complete three-part Yoga breath' described as a combination of diaphragmatic, thoracic and clavicular breathing. The inhalation starts, as Swami Niranjananda Saraswati states, with a contraction of the diaphragm, then the intercostals contract and finally the neck muscles, to fill the lungs with as much air as possible. The exhalation relaxes the diaphragm, intercostals and neck muscles.

Is this a useful breath? The thoracic and clavicular breath is an in-built emergency mechanism not to be used in daily life. The thoracic and clavicular breath kick in when the diaphragmatic breath cannot supply enough oxygen, in strenuous exercise or in fight-or-flight mode. But we do not practise Yoga in a state of emergency. All contemporary research stresses the importance of the sole diaphragmatic breath rather than a complete three-part breath. Over-breathing can cause harm, as it does in panic attacks. That is why sufferers of panic attacks are advised to breathe into a paper bag, to reduce oxygen intake. Not breathing enough is usually not an issue; it takes skilled mind control to reduce the breath.

The 'complete three-part Yoga breath' was extended into a nine-part breath. In a pranayama workshop I attended years ago, we were asked to place our hands on the body to feel the movement of the breath in all areas: (1) the abdomen, (2) the sides, (3) the lower back, (4) the chest, (5) the sides of the ribcage, (6) the upper back, (7) the clavicles, (8) under the armpits and (9) the very upper back. Even though it was called 'the complete Yoga breath', nowhere is this instructed in any traditional Indian Yoga tradition.

Using the whole lung capacity does not lead to the aim of pranayama, which is the cessation of breath.

When studying and practising the Yoga tradition over the years – the Upanishads, Patanjali, Hatha compositions and many more – I have never come across a reference to the complete three-part Yoga breath, or to the diaphragm or other breathing muscles, or to the need to fill the lungs to their fullest extent with air. What I have found are descriptions of the vayu movement, instructions to remain in the space after the vayu reverse, and kumbhaka, to stop breathing so that kundalini awakes and rises up sushumna.

The other common practice that is taught as pranayama in Western Yoga classes is 'nadi sodhana'. This is the name we gave the practice of alternate nostril breathing. 'Nadi' are the Prana conductors, and 'sodhana' means purifying. And yes, purifying the nadis is pranayama, but the term does not refer to closing one nostril. Googling 'pranayama' brings up a lot of pictures, most of practitioners closing one nostril. I have never found the term 'nostril' in any Sanskrit Hatha texts in the context of pranayama. The closest I have found is the word 'nasagra' (tip of the nose) in the instruction of padmasana (lotus seat) where the gaze is directed to the tip of the nose (HYP 1, 46). The term 'nostrils' is found in translations when the Sanskrit text speaks about either 'pingala' and 'ida' or 'surya' and 'chandra', which are terms referring to either nadis or chakras, not nostrils. I have never found the instruction of closing one nostril in any Sanskrit text.

I will discuss later why I believe that nostrils are not involved in any Hatha practice. Old paintings and sculptures of Indian Yogis in asana and meditation exist, none with a Yogi closing one nostril. That does not prove that Indian Yogis did not close their nostrils, but I feel that at least some doubt is appropriate.

We do breathe when practising pranayama. Respiration and the movement of the vayu occur in the same rhythm. The respiration in pranayama will be diaphragmatic as vayu movement has its origin in manipura, in the mid-abdomen. A thoracic breath blocks the vayu movement. Yoga beginners often cannot breathe diaphragmatically, which makes the experience of pranayama impossible for them.

The Yoga teacher training syllabus of the British Wheel of Yoga, which I taught for 20 years, teaches 'basic breathing' before proceeding to pranayama for that very reason. Nevertheless, I found through my teaching more and more that the best way to enable students to breathe diaphragmatically is by instructing pranayama. The focus on the vayu movement enables most students to remain in diaphragmatic breath.

Pranayama practice is linked with respiration, like an oar to a rowing boat. An oar is substantially different from a rowing boat, but both are needed to create a rowing experience. Diaphragmatic breathing is by nature the default respiration. Beginners who join a Yoga class in the West and whose breathing is habitually thoracic or clavicular have changed the default. Their bodies have settled to be in a state of non-stop emergency. The modern Western lifestyle is based on a state of non-stop emergency. Work life is very competitive, everyone needs to be constantly performing at a high level. Leisure activities are competitive, from sports to games. Even social life becomes a competition: Who has more friends and followers on social media? Who is more popular? People with chronic thoracic breathing do not over-breathe; their bodies have swapped diaphragmatic for thoracic breathing. The abdominal wall will be in chronic tension, which blocks the pranayama movement. Relearning free diaphragmatic breathing is needed for pranayama. Relearning breathing is best when sitting or lying and being instructed. When attempting to bring the newly gained diaphragmatic breath into asana, it often returns to thoracic and clavicular breathing as the physical movement is associated with the achievement of the outer form. To maintain the newly learned breathing in asana, as well as in all daily life, we only need to focus on breathing, not any specific technique. Our priorities need to change: the breath becomes the centre of our awareness, not the achievement of a posture or a task in life.

Practical: develop diaphragmatic breath
The easiest posture in which to regain diaphragmatic breathing is savasana. Lie on the back, place one hand on the belly and witness its rising during the inhalation and sinking during the exhalation. If this is difficult, then it helps to place a weight like a book or a Yoga gravel bag on the belly.

Note: most students are able to find the abdominal movement straight away. Some find it more difficult and need extra work, such as rhythmical contractions of the abdominal wall or detachment practices. In some cases, a teacher needs imagination to break a thoracic breathing habit. When I once tried unsuccessfully to instruct all sorts of techniques to one of my students, I placed, in desperation, a yellow crystal on her belly, and to the astonishment of everyone present, the student's belly started to rise and sink.

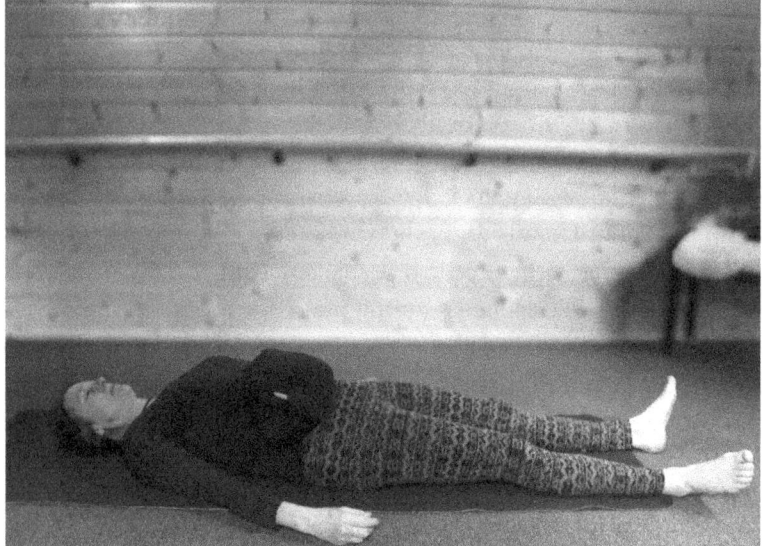

Figure 4.1 *Savasana with gravel bag on the tummy*

When free belly movement is established, sit in a comfortable upright posture. Do not try to do the 'right breath'; let it happen and witness it. That might work for a while, but when the focus drifts, the habitual thoracic breathing returns. A teacher needs to use frequent reminders and observe the breathing of the students. When practising alone, remind yourself regularly to breathe abdominally.

More complicated asana practice makes it harder to focus on the belly movement. Start with easy postures when focusing on the breath. Remind yourself that this is breathing practice, not posture practice. After some asana with the focus on the diaphragmatic breath, sit and watch. You should find the movement in the belly less effortful. At this point, we believe that we feel diaphragmatic breath, because that is what our knowledge tells us. But we cannot feel our diaphragm moving any more than we can feel our liver detoxifying.

When knowledge of your physiology is no longer interfering and you have no more inner vision of your body, then you sense a subtle expanding of the flickering aliveness from the navel centre outwards, the reverse back to the navel centre and a complete arriving. At this point, forget about diaphragmatic breathing and allow your awareness to be with the vayu movement. In that state, you have a deeper connection with your 'breathing'; you come into a stiller, deeper place where breath and focus are effortless, like entering a deeper dimension. It is like looking at a 'magic eye' 3D picture. We look at a two-dimensional image and focus. There comes a moment when you feel as if you are sucked into the picture and see the hidden three-dimensional image and connect to the deeper and subtler truth.

After a while, return intentionally to thoracic breathing and experience how you are pulled out of the deeper, subtler plane back into the outer appearance.

In my early years of teaching, I had regular one-to-one sessions with an experienced teacher. One day, she told me how astonishing she finds it when newcomers to her classes cannot even feel their diaphragm moving. I thought a lot about her statement, feeling inadequate, because I could not feel my diaphragm moving. You feel something in your abdomen, which is not a contraction of a muscle and inner organs being compressed, but you feel an expansion and drawing back of the vayu movement. This is what my teacher referred to: she actually spoke about the experience of pranayama.

Not all Western Yoga teaching reduces pranayama to an anatomical process. Swami Satyananda Saraswati's Bihar School of Yoga, which became influential in the West, has a wider view on pranayama. Swami Satyananda Saraswati tried in his teaching to connect the pranic reality with the knowledge of anatomy:

> Pranayama should not be considered as mere breathing exercises aimed at introducing extra oxygen into the lungs. Pranayama utilises breathing to influence the flow of prana in the nadis or energy channels of the pranamaya kosha or energy body. (Swami Satyananda Saraswati 1996a, p.363)

How the breathing utilizes the flow of prana in the nadis is not specified. Another of the Bihar books, *Prana Pranayama Prana Vidya*, makes a useful distinction between psychic breath and gross breath in the chapter 'Unlocking Pranamaya Kosha'. The gross breath is drawing air into the lungs and expelling it; the psychic breath is breathing connected with the psychic passage, sushumna, and the psychic centres, the chakras. That is a good pranayama definition, which is unfortunately not carried through the book. The psychic breath is still seen as an anatomical process:

> In the initial stages of psychic breathing, the only requirement is psychic awareness of the breath. That is, becoming aware of the breath without trying to affect the natural flow of the breath cycle. Once this is achieved the movement of the breath during inhalation and exhalation is to be experienced in the form of ujjayi pranayama. (Swami Niranjanananda Saraswati 2002, p.64)

Ujjayi as well as breath awareness can be applied during both respiration and pranayama; those techniques do not necessarily initiate the experience of the difference. I always felt when reading the above passage that I was being left in dark by the author about the real nature of pranayama.

We have to be a scholar and a practitioner

The Yoga compositions that we inherited from India are not philosophical statements; they are in most cases instructions, and there is a crucial difference. Philosophy, as we understand it, is a discipline established in ancient Greece (*philos* = friend; *sophia* = wisdom), working with the logical capacity of the human mind. Concepts of the nature of the universe and humanity are formulated, compared and agreed or disagreed with. A philosophical school or a religion agrees that a concept is true and formulates it in the form of dogmas, which are then believed. The main Yoga principle, on the other hand, is deactivating and stilling the mind: no thought, no logic, no concept, going beyond thought to a direct experience. Nothing needs to be believed or not believed, but a level of deeper truth is experienced.

The Indian Yoga instructions are not formulations of truth, but pointers to the direction where an experience of truth can occur. When asked what the moon is, one uses a finger to point at it. The finger is not the moon. But when following the pointing finger with the eyes, it might be possible to see the moon and experience a level of truth of the moon. Yoga instructions are not the truth; they are the pointers, invitations – when followed, truth might be experienced. An instruction without a practice is useless. When being taught that there is a force called apana moving from manipura downwards and then reversing, we are not meant to believe or disbelieve the statement, but sit down, be open-minded, follow the instructions and experience the movement. The result of the practice is not an agreeing or disagreeing with the teaching, but either having 'seen' it or not having 'seen' it. We have to be a practitioner – not just a practitioner who merely follows the instructions once and then knows it, but a practitioner who is in an ongoing process of practice to remain connected to the truth. The Yoga Sutras of Patanjali give instructions for how to reach the state of Yoga, which are then followed by the statement:

> But this practice has to be firmly grounded for a long time, without interruption and in full observance. (Patanjali 1, 14)

Simply being a practitioner does not lead to progression; we also have to be a scholar. When there is only practice, we stay 'blind' and unaware, which is common in modern Yoga when asana are watched on YouTube and imitated. With a scholarly approach, one looks at the heritage, the verses of the old Yogis, translating them, understanding them, interpreting them and then applying them in practice – otherwise, Yoga practice becomes a boring and repetitive exercise without meaning and further learning. It is unfortunate that our culture separated those two capacities – scholarship and practice – because both are needed in Yoga. We are encouraged to be either on the mat and stretching our hamstrings or sitting at a desk in an academic institution, pondering and comparing. Progress in Yoga occurs when we are scholarly practitioners or practising scholars, and these two elements need to be interwoven. Sitting at a desk all day pondering and visiting a Yoga class in the evening to unwind is also not effective. The learned knowledge is applied on the mat; the practice is a follow-on of the instructions that have been understood. I get most of my insights on my Yoga mat, but they can only happen on my mat because I have studied the heritage.

I recall working on the subject of the vayu in the Yoga teacher training course I attended. We looked at a diagram of a person with prana in the chest, apana in the pelvis, samana in the abdomen and udana in arms and legs. Our practical sessions never referred to vayu. None of us understood the relevance of the vayu teaching and, as far as I could gather, nor did the tutor. We had only been mere scholars and our practice happened unconnected to the knowledge we gained.

In the next section, I apply the scholarly approach and look at the evidence of pranayama in the old Indian Yoga compositions, to 'excavate' the message that has been covered by cultural misunderstandings and mistranslations, before applying this in practice. I hope that after this section the reader will no longer be confronted with the question 'Is this right or wrong?' or 'Do I believe this or not?' but will repond, 'Oh yes, I see this now!'

Pranayama explained in the Hatha verses

Refrain

Pranayama is not respiration, but the expansion of Prana. Pranayama is a process not in the physical body but in the pranic body. Prana is not air or breath, but life that enters each embryo and settles in the navel centre; death occurs when Prana, life, leaves.

Pranayama, the expansion of Prana, is a threefold process: (1) the expanding of Prana from its origin in the navel centre outwards; (2) the reversing of Prana back to the navel centre; and (3) the containing of Prana in the navel centre. The threefold process is called vayu, and it happens in the rhythm of the breath, but it is not breath, and it moves in the opposite direction to respiration. Vayu does not move through air tubes but through nadis. The nadis are full of impurities, and pranayama is the purification process. Once the nadis are purified, the vayu stops moving and breath ceases. Prana then remains for prolonged periods in the navel centre where it creates heat, which awakens a dormant pranic force sitting in the base chakra, kundalini. Kundalini rises in the innermost, spiritual nadi, sushumna; when it reaches the top, sahasrara, an enlightened state occurs.

The Indian Hatha Yogis of the fifth century through to the 14th century CE were not concerned with physical respiration but with pranayama, a process in pranayama kosha. The Hatha Yoga Pradipika does not work with the mental layers, but refers to Raja Yoga. The mind control of Raja Yoga and the nadi purification of Hatha Yoga go hand in hand:

> There is no Hatha without Rajayoga and no Rajayoga without Hatha. One would not succeed in practice when not practising the pair to perfection. (HYP 2, 76)

Pranayama is defined in the first six verses of chapter 2, and no physical benefits or physical body parts are mentioned. Pranayama is a process in the pranic body with the aim of purifying the nadis:

> Do that pranayama always with a sattvic (illuminated) mind so that the malas (impurities) in sushumna nadis attain purity. (HYP 2, 6)

Later in chapter 2, the eight kumbhakas are described, which are not called pranayama. Some of those practices help to establish kumbhaka, the pause after exhalation, others less so, such as hissing for cooling. Benefits mentioned for the practices called kumbhakas are not exclusively pranic. For example:

> This Sitali kumbhaka cures colic, spleen, fever, bile disorder, hunger, thirst and defeats poison. (HYP 2, 58)

The Hatha Yogis were concerned with the vayu movement and not with respiration. The entrance of vayu into the body marks the beginning of the life; the exit is death. As long as there is life, there is vayu. To assume that Prana is taken from the atmosphere into our system with each inhalation and that we use it up like petrol is used by a car is a common misunderstanding.

Pranayama is the process of clearing the nadis

The clearest, most precise definition of pranayama is given in the second chapter of the Hatha Yoga Pradipika, in verses 2–6. Below are listed the five verses in transliterated Sanskrit and their translations; I will revisit these verses in later passages of the book:

2, 2: *cale vate calam cittam nishcale nishcalam bhavet /*
yogi sthanutvam apnoti tato vayum nirodhayet //

When vata (wind) moves, citta (mind) moves, when vata is still, citta is still.
The Yogin obtains firmness (in the stillness), therefore vayu (wind) should cease.

2, 3: *yavad vayuh sthito dehe tavaj jivanamn ucyte /*
maranam tasya niskrantis tato vayum nirodhayet //

For as long as there is vayu in the body, there is said to be life.
Death is the departure of that (vayu), therefore it should be stopped.

2, 4: *malakulasu nadisu maruto naiva madhyagah /*
katham svad unmanibhavah karyuasiddhih katham bhavet //

When malakulasa (clinging obstacles) are in the nadis, marut (synonym of vayu) is not in the middle (middle nadi, sushumna), how can there be unmani (still mind), how can siddhis (special powers) be gained?

2, 5: *shuddhim eti yada sarvamnadichakram malakulasam /*
tadaiva jayate yogi pranasangrahane kshamah //

When malakulsa in the nadis become pure,
then indeed is the Yogi born to the complete access to Prana

2, 6: *pranayamam tatah kuryan nityamsattvikaya dhiya /*
atha sushumnadistha malah shuddhim prayanti cha //

Do that pranayama always with a sattvic (illuminated) mind
so that the malas (impurities) in sushumna nadis attain purity

ANALYSIS OF VERSE 2, 4
I consider this verse to be one of the most important statements for the understanding of pranayama.

When malakulasa (clinging obstacles) are in the nadis, marut (synonym of vayu) is not in the middle (middle nadi, sushumna), how can there be unmani (still mind), how can siddhis (special powers) be gained?

*malakulasu nadisu maruto naiva madhyagah /
katham svad unmanibhavah karyuasiddhih katham bhavet //*

mala = obstruction, obstacle, attachment
kulasa = clinging on to
marut = wind, synonym of vayu
naiva = not at all
madhya = middle, referring to sushumna
gah = going
katham = how
sva = one's own
unmani = still mind, synonym of samadhi
bhava = becomes
karya = having made, having done
siddhi = special ability
bhavet = becomes

Obstructions (malas) are clinging (kulasa) in the nadis. The subtle network of Prana conductors in pranamaya kosha lacks clarity. Chinese medicine came to the same insight and developed methods such as acupuncture to free blockages from the meridians. The obstructions cling (kulasa) in the nadis; they are not just blockages. They cling as if they were empowered by their own will. They prevent vayu or marut from moving freely. The vayu cannot expand fully, nor can it reverse completely; sushumna stays closed and no Prana enters sushumna.

The verse implies that the purpose of pranayama is the vayu entering and rising in sushumna; only then can there be unmani, which is one of many words used to describe the heightened state that Yoga practice is aiming for: 'Raja Yoga, samadhi, unmani, manonmani, amaratva, laya, tattva, sunya, asunya, parama pada, amanaska, avaita, niralambha, nirtanjnana, jivanamukti, sahaita and turya are all synonymous' (HYP 4, 4).

Unmani and all the other words indicate a transcended state that every human can potentially reach. When an inner purification has been achieved by a spiritual practice, that state (usually called 'enlightenment' in English) occurs. The medieval Catholic saints knew this state and reached it by prayer and moral conduct. The Buddhists reach enlightenment by meditation; so did the Rajas Yogis. The Upanishadic Jnana Yogis gained enlightenment by meditation, the Bhakti Yogis by devotion and the Hatha Yogis by purifying the pranic body through practices like pranayama. A wide spectrum of practices have been used by all sorts of different cultures; all of these practices have the potential to lead to enlightenment. Our modern Western culture is possibly one of the only cultures in human history not to acknowledge the possibility of a higher state of being – other than taller statues and greater wealth. Enlightenment is foreign to us and is often even considered to be superstition. It is ironic that the European period in history that convinced us that there is no such human possibility as enlightenment was called the 'Age of Enlightenment' – a time when the belief developed that the only way to come to any understanding is through intellectual reason. Our culture replaced the striving for enlightenment with a striving for wealth and health. The Yoga tradition, which had enlightenment as a goal, changed into a health-promoting therapy. Pranayama therefore became a technique to establish respiratory health.

Any human in any time needs to evolve towards enlightenment, whether we believe in it or not, and verse 2, 4 states that the practice of pranayama leads to enlightenment.

Practical: experience the malas

Sit and drop your centre of perception into the navel centre and refrain from thought as much as possible. Perceive the vayu movement expanding outwards from the navel centre and reversing back. Focus determinedly on the reverse: we are aiming for a movement that doesn't peter out, but accelerates back into the navel centre. With practice, you will eventually see obstructions that prevent the unobstructed flow: the nadis are full of impurities.

To accomplish the reverse of the vayu into the navel centre, it is helpful to apply a short contraction of the abdominal wall at the end of the reverse. Visualize the flow of the reverse as a stream into a 'black hole' (an event in space where matter is sucked inward). The short abdominal contraction can 'push the vayu over the edge' into the black hole. The more you are able to surrender the reversing vayu into the 'black hole', the more you feel a sensation of lightness and awareness rising from the base chakra up sushumna. More and more, you will notice that a substantial change can happen when the reverse becomes unblocked and complete; Prana reaches a deeper inner dimension.

The malas are the main culprit. The destination for each soul is to reach the state of the many names. Malas are obstacles on the path of Yoga and removing them is the goal – not by effort but by letting nature go its own way. The flow of nature is experienced by the Hatha Yogis as unobstructed vayu movement.

This is not just Hatha wisdom, but knowledge of older Yoga cultures, like the Yoga Sutras of Patanjali who formulated the same truth 1500 years ago:

> The cause of the removal of obstacles is nature (the removal happens by nature), not instigated (by an active attempt of the practitioner), like a farmer (who just removes obstructions, like shade and dryness, so that nature can grow the plants). (Patanjali 4, 3)

There are obstacles and they have to be removed; this, according to Hatha and Raja, leads to the enlightened state.

The vayu movement is the cleanser. The expansion of the vayu reaches the impure areas and the reverse can shift the impurities. Following the identification of the malas in the nadis, verse 2, 6 defines this purification process as pranayama: 'Do that pranayama always with a sattvic (illuminated) mind so that the malas (impurities) in sushumna nadis attain purity' (HYP 2, 6).

Pranayama is the practice to clear the nadis from malas.

Practical: pranayama happens by nature; it is not 'achieved'

Try to approach this practice wholeheartedly. Once you experience pranayama, it becomes an obvious process and you will no longer need to apply effort.

After asana practice, sit still in a comfortable place and position. Allow a few breaths and let the centre of perception, which usually sits in the head, drop into the navel centre. As it settles there, witness the vayu movement – the expanding from the navel centre outwards and a reversing back. The expanding could reach a long way, and the reverse could return completely to the origin of the pranic forces, but this is unlikely: the nadis are full of impurities. Look at the nature of the impurities – that which prevents the free flow – and you will discover that they have their own dynamic, like their own will; they are Ego tendencies – I hold on, I cling, I have to be in control and I do not allow aliveness to expand and flow back. Then you will know that nothing other than 'undoing' needs to be done; you do not need to interfere with the natural process.

What are these impurities?

I have often heard the interpretation that the impurities mentioned in the HYP are toxins. The anatomical body can be impure with toxins, but impurities in the pranic body are of a subtler substance. Years ago, one of my meditation teachers gave us his take on those 'impurities'. He believed the impurities are attachments, an activity of the Ego. I have worked with this idea since then. In my practice, it became clearer and clearer to me that the pranayama process is obstructed, not by an arbitrary element, such as leaves that block drains, but by my own Ego sense. There is an inner resistance coming from 'me', and that resistance clings to a non-physical aspect of me. As I gained more experience of pranayama, I realized that the reverse of the vayu has the potential to release these clinging elements, to detach them. This un-clinging is not caused by the air leaving the lungs, which is a pretty weak process. The detachment is caused by the active, powerful returning of our life force back into its origin; this loosens the malas and takes them down into the inner fire to be burned. As a result, the pranic aliveness can spread better throughout the system. Toxins in the physical body would not be released by that process.

Not only my practice but also my study of the Sanskrit verses confirmed my teacher's assumption. The Sanskrit term for impurities is 'mala kulasam'. Kulasam means 'cling', and mala is 'impurity, dust, dirt or obstacle'. Georg Feuerstein defines 'mala' in his *Encyclopedic Dictionary of Yoga* with the words:

> All spiritual traditions are agreed that the ordinary person exists in a state of impurity that prevents the dawning of real wisdom (jnana). The yogic path can be viewed as a massive self-purification. Perfect purity is equated with liberation. The Tattva-Vaishardi (IV.31) identifies the defilements as the 'causes of suffering' (kleshas) and karma. (Feuerstein 1990, p.207)

A dawning of real wisdom is not the result of reducing toxins in the body. The complete clearing of malas leads to liberation. Complete detachment leads to liberation, which is made very apparent in the Bhagavad Gita: 'Always perform your duty without attachment, attachment free performance leads to the highest state' (Bhagavad Gita 34, 19).

In the Yoga tradition, the term 'mala' is a synonym of 'klesha', the term used in Feuerstein's definition. The Patanjali Yoga Sutras define kleshas as fivefold: 'Avidhya asmita raga dvesha abhinivesha klesha' (Patanjali 2, 3).

Avidhya is ignorance, the cause of the other four defilements; asmita is me-ness, Ego, whose activity is attachment; raga is attachment in the form of desire, wanting; dvesha is attachment in the form of not wanting, being averse; abhinivesha is clinging to physical life, the ultimate attachment. The kleshas are attachments. The evidence points clearly to the truth of my teacher's statement: malas are attachments.

Where there are attachments (malas in the nadis), there is no vyana (the vayu flickering in the purified areas). Apana, prana, samana and udana cannot move in impure areas, but they can reach towards them and act as purifiers. When purified, vyana enters the nadis, resulting in the sense of life and lightness.

Attachments are formed in the mental layer, manomaya kosha; they deposit malas in the nadis system, in pranamaya kosha, which causes the physical body, annamaya kosha, to react with muscular tension and a fight-or-flight response. Any attempt to clear tensions from the muscular system does not go to the root; the purifying process needs to address the attachments located in the mental kosha and the impurities in the pranic kosha.

Refrain

Pranayama is not respiration, but the expansion of Prana. Pranayama is a process not in the physical body but in the pranic body. Prana is not air or breath, but life that enters each embryo and settles in the navel centre; death occurs when Prana, life, leaves.

Pranayama, the expansion of Prana, is a threefold process: (1) the expanding of Prana from its origin in the navel centre outwards; (2) the reversing of Prana back to the navel centre; and (3) the containing of Prana in the navel centre. The threefold process is called vayu, and it happens in the rhythm of the breath, but it is not breath, and it moves in the opposite direction to respiration. Vayu does not move through air tubes but through nadis. The nadis are full of impurities, and pranayama is the purification process. Once the nadis are purified, the vayu stops moving and breath ceases. Prana then remains for prolonged periods in the navel centre where it creates heat, which awakens a dormant pranic force sitting in the base chakra, kundalini. Kundalini rises in the innermost, spiritual nadi, sushumna; when it reaches the top, sahasrara, an enlightened state occurs.

Common techniques used to facilitate pranayama

Many techniques commonly known as 'pranayama practices' are not pranayama. Pranayama is the process of the expansion of prana, apana, samana and udana, as well as the expansion of vyana and the expansion and raising of kundalini up sushumna. Techniques we use are facilitating the Prana (life)-ayama (expansion), they are preliminary practices. The Hatha compositions do not instruct pranayama techniques (see the section 'Does Hatha Yoga instruct pranayama techniques?' below).

Most practices facilitating pranayama work with breath. The nadis are full of impurities and the vayu cannot freely expand, and this results in unsteady, uncontrolled and shallow breathing. Respiration and pranayama, being independent from each other, but moving in the same rhythm, are closely related: working with one affects the other. High airflow leads to reduced Prana; reduced airflow increases Prana expansion. Slowing respiration down and decreasing the airflow increases the power of pranayama; firing up the origin of all Prana, the navel centre slows breath and decreases air volume.

Some of the techniques we use in Yoga today were instructed in the old traditions not as pranayama, but as shatkarma, kumbhaka, mudras or even asana. Some of these techniques are wonderful, and I use them a lot as they help to build up pranic awareness.

Agni sari

Agni (agni = inner fire; sari = cascade) is one of the names of the navel centre, used when referring to the heat produced in that place. Like a real fire, agni can roar with power or be cool and weak. The intensity of the inner fire can vary a lot from person to person, and it can change in different life circumstances. Sometimes it can be very weak, sometimes stronger; through the practice of agni sari, it can become more like a 'cascade' of energy. Weak agni results in low confidence and lack of determination and discipline. Weak agni does not have the power to expand Prana outwards and reverse it back; when strengthened, we can feel a clearer and less obstructed pranayama.

Agni can be invigorated like a real fire by blowing with bellows into it. The practice is a rhythmical inwards and outwards movement of the abdominal wall when the lungs are empty. Agni sari is not a practice described in any of the well-known Hatha compositions; it must have been introduced in later times. I usually instruct agni sari as the very first practice to students who are unaware of the pranic process. It is a great method to bring awareness to the navel centre and discover the power of the origin of all life. As the abdominal contractions are applied without breath, after an exhalation, agni sari is less confusing for people who are not aware of their breathing.

> **Practical: agni sari**
> We know the abdominal space contains our guts, but agni is not in the guts; it is a subtler reality. We cannot become aware of our guts, but we can become aware of agni.

Place one hand on the tummy. Inhale, then exhale. Stop breathing; remain in the pause after the exhalation and contract the abdominal wall, and then let it go again in a relatively fast rhythm. Inwards–outwards–inwards–outwards–inwards–outwards… Stop the movement when you have to breathe again; your agni sari is followed by an inhalation. If you feel you have to gasp for air, then you have continued the abdominal contractions too long and run out of oxygen. Find a good rhythm and practise a few more rounds for up to a minute, then sit still, becoming aware of the sensation of higher intensity in the mid-abdomen and witnessing the movement outwards and backwards from there. The origin of the vayu in the mid-abdomen will feel clearer, more fiery and warm; Agni sari is the invigoration of the inner fire.

Ujjayi

This is a powerful name (ud = up, superior; jaya = conquest, success) for a powerful practice. A contraction in the throat creates a sonorous breathing sound. The breath – the bodily rhythm, the waving of the conductor's arms to the orchestra (see the analogy in Chapter 3) – is directed and becomes clearer and more tangible. Ujjayi is like the baton a conductor uses to make the arm movements more visible. Applying ujjayi also binds the focus better to the breathing rhythm. I often compare ujjayi to a saddle: the rider is the focused mind, and the horse is the breath. Focusing on the breath leads frequently to a loss of attention; the rider falls off the horse. Placing a saddle on the horse gives the rider a steadier seat. With ujjayi, the vayu reaches further, is less likely to peter out and has more strength to break through impurities. Ujjayi is instructed in the HYP and the Gheranda Samitha (GS) as one of the kumbhakas.

Practical: ujjayi

Contract the throat slightly to breathe with a sonorous sound. Do not make yourself hoarse – ujjayi is effort-free breathing despite being powerful. The best way is to listen to someone breathing in ujjayi and then imitate it. If you find it difficult, then practise ujjayi first on the exhalation only: open your mouth and imagine you are steaming up a mirror. A sound should occur; close the mouth when you feel confident, maintaining the sound, and eventually include the inhalation. Direct your breath to areas in your pranic body that need attention. It is like pressing a thumb on the end of a hosepipe; the restriction causes the water to reach further and the aim is more precise.

Tadagi

Tadagi (deep pool, water well) is not found in the HYP, but in the later GS it is listed under 'mudras'. Just one verse is dedicated to tadagi: 'In pashimottanasana make the belly hollow like a well...this is tadagi the destroyer of old age and death' (GS 3, 61).

Tadagi is a beautiful practice. Ujjayi is a prerequisite for the effectiveness of the practice. The abdomen is drawn inwards with a long and complete ujjayi exhalation, creating a hole, like a well. One should remain in the abdominal contraction for a while without breathing to awaken the power in the navel centre, the pranic store. It differs from agni sari in that it is done with the breath, with a long complete pranic reverse. It is a step up from agni sari and more powerful.

Practical: tadagi

Apply ujjayi, the throaty sound, and draw the abdominal wall deep into the middle of the abdomen with each pranic reverse. Dig a deep hole, and when you arrive at the bottom of your 'well', stay there. Keep the power and tone in the abdomen but relax the rest of the body. You will find that your shoulders, chest, back muscles and thighs have tightened up. Relax the abdominal wall before the pranic expansion. Imagine you are digging a well: you do not only want to shovel loose earth out of the hole, but with each breath you want to dig deeper into the hard soil, loosening areas you have not loosened before. After a few rounds, return to pure observation and perceive the subtle movement of the vayu. In particular, the reverse will be more complete, higher in clarity, slightly less blocked; your inner fire has flared up.

Kabalabhati

Commonly known today as a pranayama practice, kapalabhati (kapala = head; bhati = shining; kapalabhati = particular form of penance) is not mentioned in the HYP at all. The GS lists kapalabhati under shatkarmas, which are physical cleansing practices, preliminary to Yoga, that are only needed when the body is full of phlegm and mucus. As a shatkarma, kapalabhati works in the head area, as the name indicates, and clears the sinuses. Through contractions of the abdominal wall in the rhythm of the breath, the airflow through the nostrils is accelerated, which allows mucus to exit from the sinuses – basically, blowing the nose. A nasal sound is heard with each exhalation. The same practice can be taken lower into the throat, which is also a shatkarma, loosening mucus in the throat. Both of these variations cleanse the physical body, but through the rhythmic abdominal movement, the inner fire, agni, is invigorated, which makes it possible to remain a long time in kumbhaka, the still phases after the complete vayu reverse, after the practice. When the same practice is lowered into the belly, it works predominantly on the pranic level. The abdominal wall contracts with each pranic reverse, but there is no nasal or throaty sound. The abdominal movement is much more intense in this variation, and it can feel as if the navel centre pulsates. When switching to the belly version, the elongated kumbhaka does not take place straight away, but pranayama can be felt better. Practitioners who are used to the nasal kapalabhati will find the belly variation strong and cannot initially sustain the practice for very long.

Practical: kapalabhati

In the head: Take a tissue and blow your nose in a fast rhythmical way, first through one nostril only, then the other, then both. Your nostrils narrow, the airflow increases and accelerates; your focus will be in the head and you will hear a nasal sound with each exhalation. Avoid a sound with the inhalation. Check whether your abdomen moves the right way, inwards with an exhalation and outwards during the inhalation. Start the practice with long enough pauses between the breaths to not get confused. Once you feel confident with the movement, you can speed up, but avoid any effort. You strain your breath if a strong thoracic inhalation follows the end of the practice. You can start with 20–50 contractions and build up to 300 over the course of weeks or months of daily practice. When you finish one round, remain in a beautiful long, still place. When the breath returns, it is of subtler nature.

In the throat: Lower the practice to the throat as if clearing the throat in a fast rhythmical manner. Don't overdo the throat practice; if mucus loosens, it will usually happen during the first 20 breaths. Spit the mucus into a tissue and return to the sense of the subtle vayu movement.

In the belly: Finally, drop your awareness into the belly, widen the nostrils to reduce the airflow, lengthen the back of the neck and bring the chin closer to the chest. Imagine you are flattening the voice-box down from above and place the tip of the tongue to the roof of the mouth. Try not to be aware that you have a nose, throat and respiration; connect to the rhythmic belly movement. Imagine you are sitting in the navel centre and experience a strong pulsation from there. No nasal sound and very little other sound is heard. The navel centre pulsates as if it is the heart of the pranic body. There is power and strength, but no force. There is movement in the abdomen, but the rest of the body stays upright and stable. When finishing the contractions, stay alert and focus on the subtle but powerful movement in the belly, an intense sense of pranic expansion and reverse, as if no respiration at all is taking place. Your expanding vayu can feel unlimited, unlike inhalation which cannot go beyond full lungs. The reversing vayu becomes stronger and carries on and on until it eventually reaches its destination and there is a still pause, the kumbhaka, which, after a few circles of pranayama, will become predominant. Kapalabhati is not pranayama but facilitates it.

Bastrika

Bastrika (little bag, bellows) is listed in the HYP under the practices called kumbhaka; it is the kumbhaka with the highest praise, and the practice is mentioned again in chapter 3 as a means to awaken kundalini. The practitioner is instructed to fill (purachet) the sun (surya), meaning the inner fire, manipura chakra, with wind (pavana, a synonym of vayu), like the bellows of a blacksmith (HYP 2, 62–63). This indicates a short, strong and pointed gush of vayu back into the inner fire, which happens during the exhalation. In this respect, it is like the fourth variation of kapalabhati: it includes a short, strong and pointed gush of vayu outwards during the inhalation. A nasal sound is heard during the inward and outward movement. It is advised to apply padmasana, the full lotus position, during the practice, because this is the most stable postion to prevent the whole body moving. Bastrika is a powerful practice and should be practised with care: it should not be practised with any form of heart problem, respiratory or abdominal disease, or ante- or postnatally. With kapalabhati, there is no upper limit on the number of breaths, but bastrika should not exceed 50 breaths in one round. The HYP names the benefits of bastrika as dosha regulation (the Ayurvedic body types), an increase of the inner fire, the destruction of impurities in the nadis, as well as the breaking of knots in sushumna, granthis and the awakening of kundalini (HYP 2, 65–66).

> **Practical: bastrika**
> Bastrika should not be attempted without the help of an experienced teacher. Practise kapalabhati until you feel confident with it and have built up the number of breaths in kapalabhati to 300. Practise isolating the different vayus (revisit the section on vayus in Chapter 3) and settle on a clear, distinct samana vayu. Sit upright, ideally in a full lotus; draw the chin down to the chest and bring your focus to the navel centre. Expand and reverse the samana vayu, first slowly, and then stronger and shorter like the bellows of a blacksmith. Start with no more than 20 breaths and monitor yourself well after the first round to see whether a repeat is advisable. Do not repeat if you feel light-headed or your pulse is faster; these symptoms will settle over time with short practice spells. You should be able to prolong the kumbhaka without effort. If you want to take the practice further, you will need to become adept in the bandha practice (see Chapter 5).

Bhramari

Bhramari (bee) is listed under kumbhakas in the HYP. It is simple, straightforward and suitable for everyone. 'Making a noise like a bee' (HYP 2, 68) is the instruction – humming. It is amazing how much the exhalation and with it, the reverse of the vayu can elongate when humming. The vibration of the hum steadies and smooths the exhalation and the vayu reverse. A shortened vayu reverse is caused by impurities (malas) sitting in the nadis. Completing the vayu reverse is a detaching process that purifies the nadis, which is encouraged by the vibration. On the physical level, the humming contributes to the relaxation of all breathing muscles.

Practical: bhramari

First use a little technique to learn how incomplete your exhalation/vayu reverse is. Breathe in and then out, and stop the exhalation at the point you feel the impulse for inhaling. Without inhaling, open your mouth and blow. A lot more air is leaving the respiratory system. Realize that you do not complete your exhalation; recognize the necessity to elongate it. Next, sit upright and watch your breathing: how long is the exhalation? Now start humming with every exhalation, and you will be able to detect how much longer and more complete it becomes. When you stop the hum, stay seated and watch the breath; the exhalation remains longer and you might sense a less restricted drop right into the navel centre.

Simbhasana

This practice is, as the name says (simbha = lion; asana = posture), an asana, described in most Hatha compositions in the first chapter. It is one of the seated asana, one of the four most valuable in HYP, which does not satisfy our expectations of a 'strong stretch'. It is nevertheless very satisfying on the pranic level. I have confused many experienced students when teaching simbhasana in the context of pranayama, but it is a very powerful technique to facilitate pranayama. Not everyone likes simbhasana: it can be intimidating to utter a strong roaring sound, like a lion. The HYP (chapter 1, 52–54) suggests siddhasana, which is the number-one asana, the best of all, as the seat for simbhasana. 'Always practice siddhasana, it cleanses the impurities from the 72000 nadis' (HYP 1, 41).

Not much more is said about simbhasana, apart from gazing at the tip of the nose, controlling the mind and opening the mouth. We can assume the roaring with an exhalation would have been instructed because of the name of the practice. The effect of simbhasana is described as the accomplishment of the bandhas, which will occur when the vayu reverse has broken through impurities and becomes complete.

Breaking through impurities is caused by that powerful vayu reverse. It is a wonderful practice to apply or teach when the focus drifts away and fatigue fogs the mind. I often teach it after lunch on pranayama days.

Blockages and impurities are removed by simbhasana, the vayu flows more freely, the reverse is more complete, and kumbhaka, the pause after the exhalation, is prolonged, which is the prerequisite for the bandhas to occur.

Practical: simbhasana

Sit in siddhasana, placing the left heel to the perineum and the right foot on top of the left ankle; if possible, touch the heels to the middle of the pelvis to create a circuit from the legs to sushumna. If your knees are not on the floor, sit on a block. Be upright along the central axis. Prior to simbhasana, place the hands on the knees, keep the back of the neck long, open the mouth wide, stretch the tongue out and continue to breathe as before. The mouth should open enough to feel a stretch across the cheeks. Lengthen the tongue down towards the collarbones so far that the stretch reaches far back into the mouth. Turn the eye gaze upwards to the place the eyebrows meet, shambhavi mudra, and continue breathing. Remain like this for a few breaths and then release. For complete simbhasana, inhale, lift the arms up to the ceiling, exhale, mouth open, tongue out, eyes turned up, roar as loud as you can, and lower your arms and head to the floor. Continue the roaring as long as possible, drawing the abdominal wall inwards. At the very end of the exhalation, close the mouth, place the tongue back to the lower jaw, remain in the pause after the exhalation and allow a powerful 'sucking-in sensation' from the navel centre. Relax the rest of the body. When you need to breathe again, release the abdominal wall and sit up. Allow a few breaths before repeating the process two more times. Then sit still and focus on the pranic movement. Not only will you feel the vayu movement more distinctly, but you will also experience a better completion of the vayu reverse, as if the vayu was disappearing into the depth of the navel centre, and as a result feel a lightness moving up through the central axis; bandhas can occur.

Viloma

I have not found any reference to viloma (vi = apart, away; loma = hair; against the grain) in Hatha compositions. The Bihar School, founded by Swami Satyananda Saraswati, teaches viloma without referencing it, and internet descriptions of viloma also do not indicate where the different teachers got the practice from. I believe it is not a classical practice and assume it is a creation of Swami Satyananda Saraswati. As the name says, it goes against the grain. We are aiming for a smooth breath, and viloma is an interruption of the smooth flow. There are three kinds: the inhalation can be interrupted, the exhalation can be interrupted or both can be interrupted. Applying the interruptions, one gains awareness and control of the breathing. The practice unblocks and purifies the nadis, resulting in a smoother breath.

Practical: viloma

Start the viloma practice when you are comfortable with ujjayi; viloma without ujjayi is difficult.

Begin with interruption of the inhalation. Imagine you are walking up a ladder to the top of a big slide, interrupting the inhalation on each rung of the ladder, then slide down on the exhalation. Don't strain, but build up the number of steps up. Continue for about one minute and then allow a quiet period to see whether the inhalation and with it the expansion of Prana has gained a higher degree of smoothness.

Then interrupt the exhalation only. Imagine you take an elevator up to the top of a multistorey building and walk down the steps. Do not strain but build up the number of interruptions gradually. In a quiet period afterwards, monitor the smoothness of the exhalation and with it the reverse of Prana.

Proceed to double viloma. Interrupt inhalation and exhalation. Imagine you take steps up a mountain and steps back down the other side. Afterwards pause and sit still to enjoy the freer flow.

Ratio breathing

When I was training, ratio breathing was the main so-called 'pranayama technique'. Numbers were given to train the phases of the breath into a pattern. We were given Sanskrit names for the different ratios, which must have been created by some Western practitioners; those terms are not found in the Hatha tradition. The numbers would go up with practice as a higher lung capacity was reached. Everyone can practise ratio breathing as much as they want, but this is not Yoga or pranayama. There is no mention of it in the Yoga tradition. Pranayama is the removal of impurities and is aiming for a free flow of life force, not a forceful elongation and holding of the breath.

When discussing ratio breathing, one of my students asked whether control of the breath would not break through the impurities. She is right, but control of ratio breathing forces the phases into an intended pattern. The control in pranayama is applied to the obstructions; they are loosened by the controlled mind and 'breath' to bring the movement into a free, unobstructed flow, as nature intends. We apply control not to do but to undo.

Nadi sodhana

Alternate nostril breathing is usually called 'nadi sodhana' (nadi = Prana conductor; sodhana = purification). 'Purification of the nadis' is indeed what pranayama is all about, but not with a closed nostril. I am pretty sure that the alternate nostril breath is based on a translation mistake, which I will discuss in detail in the next section. Instructions in the Hatha texts that are translated to the English 'close your left or right nostril' do not use a Sanskrit word for 'nostrils', but 'ida' and 'pingala', the names of the two main nadis besides sushumna. Those two nadis are not in the anatomical body, but in the pranic body, and they have no relation to nostrils. Ida and pingala reach up from muladhara chakra to ajna chakra where they merge. Nostrils, on the other hand, are the end of the respiratory tubes.

Hatha Yoga had basically become extinct after the British takeover of the Indian subcontinent (see the section 'The historical journey of pranayama from Hatha to modern Yoga' in Chapter 2). Yoga came to the West, where it received a Western interpretation, and that interpretation returned to India. The last time I travelled in India a few years ago, I asked in most hotels or hostels if they had Yoga classes. Most had, but all of the teachers came from England. It seems that many Indians learn Yoga from British teachers and do not visit their own heritage themselves. The British Wheel of Yoga used to run annual national training weeks for Yoga teachers for further learning. I was a tutor on some of these events and was astonished to meet Indian Yoga teachers travelling from India to attend. When I expressed my astonishment, they told me that the place to learn Yoga nowadays is Britain. But British Yoga is based mostly on an anatomical understanding.

In Iyengar's *Light on Yoga*, the picture of him practising nadi sodhana shows him closing alternate nostrils. When describing the effect of nadi sodhana, he refers to it in anatomical terms: 'The blood vessels receive a larger amount of oxygen in Nadi Sodhana than in normal breathing, so that one feels refreshed and the nerves are calmed and purified' (Iyengar 1991, p.374).

Iyengar was trained by his teacher to bring Yoga to the West, so Western terminology seemed appropriate to him. Krishnamacharya, his teacher, did not pass on the 'esoteric' knowledge that has no equivalent in Western thinking.

Iyengar's statement claims that more oxygen in the blood calms the nerves, which can be explained scientifically, but breathing slowly through one nostril does not increase oxygen. He also followed the 20th-century misunderstanding that nadis are nerves, when he says that the 'nerves are calmed and purified'.

I do believe that alternate nostril breathing is a myth. People like it; it calms, it is gentle, and the focus is settled on the breath and mind, and it is therefore stilling. I often think that the love of nadi sodhana might originate from the desire to practise serious Yoga without putting effort into it. I personally have never felt much benefit from it. However, if you like alternate nostril breathing and feel you benefit from it, continue to practise it, but be aware it may not be classic pranayama.

Does Hatha Yoga instruct pranayama techniques?
What are the instructions of the classical Hatha Yoga tradition?

Earlier in this chapter, the first six verses of chapter 2 of the HYP were discussed. Verse 1 reminds us that asana need to be accomplished and a good diet established, and that pranayama is to be learned from a guru. Verses 2–5 explain that the nadis are full of impurities and need to be purified to reach an enlightened state. Verse 6 concludes the paragraph with the statement that pranayama needs to be practised to purify the nadis. That is the Hatha Yogis' summary of pranayama, not the introduction.

I have always been taught that pranayama is a collection of those techniques, which I have described above. The HYP nevertheless defines pranayama as follows:

> Pranayama is said to have three elements, rechaka (expand out) puraka (fill in), and kumbhaka (literally: pot, here referring to the pause after the exhalation). (HYP 2, 71)

Pranayama is not a collection of techniques but a process with three elements:

- Rechaka is the expansion of the vayu out of manipura, which happens during inhalation.
- Puraka is the 'filling in' or reversing of the vayu to manipura, which happens during the exhalation.
- Kumbhaka is the active stillness after the vayu reverse, when sushumna is opening.

In the second half of verse 71, Swatmarama defines kumbhaka as follows:

> Kumbhaka has two ways, sahita and kevala. (HYP 2, 71)

Sahita (= coming together with) kumbhaka is the incomplete kumbhaka. The pause after the reverse of the vayu (exhalation) is eventually followed by the expansion (inhalation). Kevala (= only, alone) is when the still pause stands alone, and is not followed by the expansion of vayu. Both kumbhakas follow the 'exhalation'; sahita kumbhaka is not fully complete, but with practice, it will eventually lead to kevala kumbhaka, as Swatmarama explicates:

> The practice of sahita is done so long till kevala occurs. (HYP 2,72)

Most Yoga teachers, including me, were taught that Yoga breath is categorized into four, not three phases:

- puraka, inhalation

- antara kumbhaka, holding the breath after the in-breath
- rechaka, exhalation
- bahir kumbhaka, holding the breath after the exhalation.

I believe that textual evidence as well as practical experience allows me to question this teaching. I believe the reason for this fourfold concept lies in the incorrect equation of pranayama with respiration.

Nowhere in the Hatha tradition is there found a fourfold distinction into puraka, antara kumbhaka, rechaka and bahir kumbhaka. I believe this category was created by Western Yoga teachers in the same way as the 'three-part full Yoga breath', and that a misinterpretation of the pranayama process took place. I am fully aware that the following statements are controversial, but I would appreciate the reader taking time to try to follow my train of thought and engage in the suggested practices to see where I am coming from and give the understanding of pranayama a fresh new start.

The verses instruct **rechaka** (expanding outwards); I assume this means the vayu expanding from the manipura outwards, which happens during the inhalation. The Western interpretation of rechaka is expelling air out of the lungs; 'outwards' and 'breath' are thought to indicate exhalation.

The next step is **puraka** (drawing/filling in); I assume this means the vayu filling into manipura, which happens during the exhalation. The modern interpretation of puraka is drawing air into the lungs, because 'inwards' and 'breath' is thought to be inhalation. What moves in the pranayama process is vayu (apana, prana, samana, udana), not air. Vayu moves in the opposite direction to airflow in breathing.

In my practice, I clearly feel an expansion from the navel centre outwards and a reversal back into the navel centre followed by a still phase. Not only do I feel this, but all of those I teach and have taught feel it too. The first instruction I give beginner students is to focus on a movement in the abdominal area of expanding outwards during the inhalation and reversing inwards during the exhalation, which makes sense to everyone. I relate the old Indian mythology of the creation of the universe. Brahman, the universal consciousness, breathes in and as such the universe expands, as we know it from the theory of the big bang. During the exhale of Brahman, all is drawn back into its origin. That mythology shows what we all experience: an expanding outward movement, rechaka, during the inhalation and a drawing back inwards, puraka, during the exhalation.

The HYP names only three elements for the pranayama process, not four, as does Patanjali (see the section 'Pranayama as described in Patanjali 2, 49–52' below): the expansion of vayu, rechaka, the reverse of vayu, puraka, and the still space of kumbhka. There is no antara or bahir kumbhaka, just kumbhaka, the third element of pranayama. Kumbhaka comes after puraka. That is the sequence indicated, first rechaka, then puraka, then kumbhaka. If rechaka was the exhalation and puraka the inhalation, then the pause, kumbhaka, would take place with full lungs after the inhalation. I believe that most Yoga practitioners would agree with me that kumbhaka is a phenomenon occurring *after* the exhalation.

My suspicion first arose when I trained as a Yoga teacher; the course was very strong on safety. We had to learn all possible conditions the students might have and how to modify practices for different conditions. For each practice, we had to name precautions, prohibitions and modifications. We learned numerous precautions and prohibitions for 'antara kumbhaka'. Anyone with heart disease, high blood pressure, eye conditions such as glaucoma or detached retina, pregnancy, anxiety or depression should refrain from the practice. Why, I wondered, is there a Yoga practice that is potentially so dangerous? My answer today is that antara kumbhaka is not a Yoga practice! I know of only one reason to practise holding the breath with full lungs and that is for diving training. There is only one kumbhaka, which initially comes in the form of sahita, the incomplete kumbhaka; breathing resumes after a while. When accomplished in pranayama, the sahita kumbhaka turns into kevala kumbhaka, the prolonged state of no breath. Yogis have been known to stop breathing for hours. This is definitely impossible when one holds the breath with full lungs. Ask someone to breathe in and hold the breath and they will tell you that this is an unpleasant experience. Train someone in pranayama and they will relatively soon come to the point of remaining without breath after the exhalation for a short time; most students refer to this experience with the words 'that is lovely'.

Let's conclude. There are three phases of pranayama:

- rechaka, the expansion of the vayu from manipura outwards
- puraka, the drawing of the vayu back into manipura

- kumbhaka, the vayu arriving back in the mid-abdomen and remaining.

Kevala kumbhaka is the accomplishment of pranayama: no more breath after the completed vayu reverse, no more vayu movement. At that point, kundalini awakes and moves up sushumna. That is the aim of pranayama.

Nowhere in the Hatha tradition have I found the terms 'bahir' (outwards) and 'antara' (inwards) connected with the word 'kumbhaka'.

From kumbhaka one can gain abilities, control and insight, crucial points the yogic development: 'There is nothing difficult to obtain in the three worlds; by the competence of kevala kumbhaka, all is possible' (HPY 2, 74).

Pranayama, as described in the HYP, is simply the focus on an inner movement and the attempt to allow it to move without interference.

Practical: kumbhaka

With your focus on the navel centre, experience the movement of pranayama. If the pranic body was free from impurities, then the vayu, the lightness and awareness would shift unobstructed outwards, expanding into wide open space, like the expansion of the universe. In the same way, the reverse of the vayu would flow unobstructed on and on and would arrive without hesitation in the navel entre. The kumbhaka at the end of the reverse would elongate as fewer impurities remain. Visualize the navel centre as the 'heart of the pranic body'. The physical heart pumps blood around the whole body, supplying each cell with oxygen. When the blood reverses, it carries carbon dioxide to be discarded. In the same way, the vayu spreads from the navel centre through the system. The reverse loosens unwanted attachments and impurities, and discards them into the inner fire – the process of purification. That is pranayama; it happens from within and all the practitioner needs to do is let the natural process happen, not obstruct it, undoing the efforts created by the Ego. Watch this process; surrender into the process. Nature knows what needs to happen, but our small mind thinks it knows better. Detach from the process: just witness and let go. Kumbhaka will gradually appear.

Modern Yoga instructs many practices classified as pranayama (see the section 'Common techniques used to facilitate pranayama' above). Are any of those based on the classic Hatha tradition?

Later in chapter 2 of the HYP (48–70), eight kumbhakas are described, but they are not called pranayama. They are called 'kumbhaka' and some of them help the practitioner to reach a more prolonged kumbhaka.

The term 'kumbhaka' is used in a twofold way in the HYP, not only as the still space after the vayu reverse, but also as a name for the practices listed in 2, 48–70 (see Feuerstein 1990, under 'kumbhaka').

Sanskrit terms, when they appear in different contexts, can have different meanings; a native speaker would not be bewildered by this. Sanskrit is a language with a particularly wide range of meanings for each word, but multiple meanings of words occur in all languages. A non-native English speaker might know the word 'party', a jolly social gathering, and the word 'gate', an entrance. They would be confused to find that the term 'partygate' is used to describe the UK political scandal following a breach of COVID restrictions and not the gate to a social gathering.

There are many other Sanskrit examples causing regular confusion, like the word 'karma', which means 'action'. It can be used in profane contexts, any activity such as cooking a meal, and is also used as a philosophical concept describing the results of one's actions, which affect their next incarnation. The word 'Atman' as we know it from the Bhagavad Gita and the Upanishads indicates the inner Self, identical to Brahman. The word can plainly mean 'self' and can be found in everyday contexts like 'He himself (Atman) went hunting in the forest'. 'Kumbhaka' means 'pot', something that has the property of containing. Kumbhaka can be the pot that contains our mangos, or a place where the vayu is contained, or a term holding a number of the practices together.

After the HYP defines pranayama as the purification of the nadis in the first six verses of the second chapter, instructions follow.

Verse 7

baddhapadmasano yogi pranamcandrena purayet, dharayitva yathasakti bhuyah suryenarecayet.

The yogi applying baddhapadmasana (lotus seat) purayet (draws in) prana from candra (moon), dharayitva (having held), recayet (expands) into surya (sun). (HYP 2, 7)

Verses 2, 7–8, are commonly translated to describes a practice resembling what we call alternate nostril breathing.

The translation of Pancham Sinh (2014) of HYP verse 7 reads:

> Sitting in padmasana posture the Yogi should fill in the air through the left nostril; and, keeping it confined according to one's ability, it should be expelled through the right nostril.

Pancham Sinh translates the word 'Prana' with 'air', the word 'candra' with 'left nostril' and the word 'surya' with 'right nostril'.

The Adyar Library translation (Swami Svatmarama 1972) reads:

> The Yogin assuming Padmasana should draw the Prana through the moon [i.e. Ida or the left nostril] and, having retained it as long as possible, should then exhale it through the Sun [i.e. Pingala or the right nostril].

That is more precise, but 'ida' is equated with 'left nostril' and 'expanding the vayu' is translated as 'exhale', but happens during the inhalation.

What does verse 7 really instruct? It gives the instruction to apply baddhapadmasana, the lotus seat with arms wrapped around the back to hold on to the feet, a still, seated posture. Pranic force should be drawn in from candra, the moon. That is the reverse of the vayu from the moon back into manipura. In the Hatha context, candra refers either to bindu, the origin of creation at the back of the head, or to ida, the left side of the pranic body, not to a nostril. Surya, the sun in the Hatha context, refers either to 'inner sun', 'inner fire' in manipura or to pingala, the right side of the pranic body, not to a nostril. Verses 2, 9 onwards use the terms ida and pingala instead of candra and surya in the same context. That indicates that 'candra' in verse 7 means 'ida', the left side of the pranic body, and 'surya' means pingala, the right side of the pranic body.

The instruction of verse 7 appears to mean to apply baddhapadmasana and reverse Prana from the left side only; remain in kumbhaka, then expand into the right side.

Verse 8

pranam suryena cakrasya purayet udaram sanai, vidhivat kumbhakam krtva punas candrena recayet.

Draw in (purayet) slowly by surya chakra (sun chakra) prana to the belly (udara), kumbhaka according to instructions (vidhivat), then recayet (expanded) into candra. (HYP 2, 8)

Pancham Sinh (2014):

Then, drawing in the air through the right nostril slowly, the belly should be filled, and after performing kumbhaka as before, it should be expelled slowly through the left nostril.

As in verse 7, Singh translates the term 'Prana' as 'air'. He translates 'surya chakra' as 'left nostril'. Here is a difference to verse 7 where the word 'surya' is used without 'chakra'. In verse 7, we had assumed surya to mean the right side of the pranic body, pingala. 'Surya chakra' is referring to a whirling condensed pranic event, a chakra, the sun chakra, manipura. The pranic force which had been expanded into the right side is now drawn in by the manipura chakra. This conclusion is confirmed by the following term 'udaram' – 'to the abdomen'. The Sanskrit 'suryena' appears in the grammatical form of an instrumentalis (a grammatical form that indicates that the word, here sun, has the meaning of being the instrument of an action, here: 'by the sun', the sun is the cause of the action), meaning it is the manipura by which the action of drawing is performed. This centre has the active power to accelerate the Prana flow back to its origin. Pancham Sinh sees surya chakra (right nostril) and udara as two different things. It is not clear what he thinks should be filled into the belly; the air entering the nostril does not go into the belly. Surya chakra and udaran are one and the same in the verse; it actively draws Prana, suryena, back into itself, udaram.

When Prana has entered manipura, kumbhaka should be applied in the way it was previously instructed, which is after the reverse of the vayu; then it is expanded into candra, the left side of the pranic body, not as in Panchan Sinh's translation which reads: 'expel air through the right nostil'.

The translation of the Adyar Library (Swami Svatmarama 1972) resembles Pancham Sinh's:

> Inhaling the Prana through the Pingala, the interior should be filled. Performing kumbhaka as prescribed, it should be then exhaled through Ida.

But Prana is not inhaled or exhaled, and ida and pingala are not nostrils!

To conclude, the instructions of 2, 7–8 are not describing alternate nostril breathing, but the process of pranayama as analysed above, with the vayu flow alternating between the right and the left side of the pranic body. From candra, the left side of the pranic body, the vayu is drawn in by the navel centre and kept there, then the vayu expands into surya, the right side of the pranic body; then manipura draws the vayu back into itself, kumbhaka occurs and the vayu is expanded into candra, the left side. We are then back at the beginning: the circle is closed.

This text analysis might be confusing and complicated, but it will seem much clearer and easier in the practice.

Practical: 'nadi sodhana' as really instructed

Sit and follow with unwavering concentration the movement of the vayu.

Apply a straight seated position, with an upright pelvis that tilts neither forwards nor backwards. Experience the movement of the vayu as it expands from the navel centre outwards and reverses back. The HYP tells us that the reverse happens by surya chakra; this inner fire has the power to actively draw the vayu back inwards, if we don't block it. Imagine the navel centre being a strong magnet, which is turned on as soon as the expanding vayu turns to reverse.

That is all the verses 2, 7–8 instruct with a small addition, the swinging of the focus on the vayu from side to side. Follow the reverse from the left side back to the navel centre, then remain in kumbhaka. Let the focus accompany the next expansion to the right side. Reverse from the right, allowing a strong shift into the navel centre. Remain in kumbhaka until the next expansion and follow it to the left side. One circle is done; repeat the process. If you enjoy the practice, continue as long as you want.

If my interpretation is right, then the question would arise: why move the focus from side to side? It is not the reverse on its own that purifies the nadis; it is the focus, the controlled mind, accompanying the vayu. Controlling the mind to remain sharply focused on the vayu movement is very difficult. As Yoga teachers, we know that when we ask students to focus on one hip and one shoulder, they find it too difficult as they can only focus on one or the other. Only a very controlled mind is able to 'see' the whole of the inner space all at once. It is easier and therefore more effective to purify the nadis on one side and then the other.

Passages on pranayama in the other Hatha compositions agree with the HYP. The 300-year-younger Gheranda Samitha (GS) describes pranayama in the fifth chapter. This chapter discusses first a good place for the practice, a suitable time and the best food to eat during the period of the practices, before instructions follow, which are headed 'Purifications of Nadis': 'atha nadi shuddhih' – 'now comes the purification of the nadis' (GS 5, 33).

Pranayama in the GS is also defined as nadi purification. The Sanskrit nadi shuddhih in the GS does not refer to closing alternate nostrils.

Verse 35 states, as in HYP 2, 3, that marut (synonym of vayu) cannot enter the nadis due to impurities (malakulasa). Therefore, pranayama is needed. The passages that follow describe a cleansing with mantra and colour visualization – a Hatha technique that must have developed in the period between HYP and the GS. Then follows a statement in perfect agreement with the HYP:

> draw in (into manipura) vayu from candra (left side)...kumbhaka (remain)...expand vayu to suryu (right side). (GS 5, 39–40)

Likewise, the same process is described in the Shiva Samitha in chapter 3, verses 22 onwards, using the same terminology.

The alternate nostril breath, which we call nadi sodhana, is one of the most common 'pranayama' practices taught in modern classes, and I believe the teaching is based on mistranslation. I have attended classes and workshops where pranayama was defined as the ability to increase sensitivity to the airflow through the nostrils. One teacher equated the process of gently closing and opening the nostrils to the skill of playing a musical instrument, and I remember, being a musician myself, feeling this analogy was a bit far-fetched.

The eight kumbhakas

After the description of pranayama at the beginning of chapter 2 in the HYP there follows a section on physical cleansing that should precede any Yoga practice if needed:

> If there is excess of fat or phlegm in the body the shatkarmas (shat = six; karma = action) should be performed first. (HYP 2, 21)

The shatkarmas (six actions) are techniques to clean the bowels, nose, stomach and sinuses. Excess phlegm and fat can be reduced by the shatkarmas in order to become ready for the Yoga journey. Shatkarmas work on the physical body. After the shatkarma instructions there follow verses praising pranayama, picking up the line again from the beginning of chapter 2: pranayama conquers the fear of death (HYP 2, 39) by the marut (vayu) being led in the middle (sushumna) (HYP 2, 40). The opening of sushumna is a result of the purification of the nadis (HYP 2, 41). The result of marut in sushumna is mental stillness (manonmani) (HPY 2, 42), a synonym of unmani (HYP 2, 3).

Verse 43 links the pranayama summary to the section of the eight kumbhakas:

> Those gain perfection of that (manonmani), who do the kumbhakan, and are knowledgable of the process. By the process of kumbhaka siddhis (special powers) are obtained. (HYP 2, 43)

The term 'kumbhaka' is used here in its plural form 'kumbhakan', the kumbhakas. When referring to the stillness after the vayu reverse, kumbhaka is always singular.

Kumbhakas do help to perfect the state of manonmani, and are practised for the attainment of special powers, the siddhis, which are all sorts of accomplishments. The kumbhakas are not classified as pranayama practices and are not said to purify the nadis.

Verses 45-47 instruct the application of the three bandhas during the practice of the kumbhakas, at the end of puraka, the drawing-in of the vayu after the exhalation. This is another statement showing how we mistakenly have turned the pranayama phases around. The bandhas are certainly applied after the reverse of the vayu, after the exhalation, which is puraka, not the filling of the lungs with air (for more on bandhas, see Chapter 5).

Eight kumbhakas are listed (HYP 2, 44 onwards).

Suryabhedana (surya = sun; bhedana = penetration) is not one of the practices we see often taught in modern Yoga. This practice, the penetrating of the sun, refers to manipura chakra in this context. In the description of this kumbhaka, we can see all the inconsistencies caused by translation, which I have discussed above, all stemming from the identification of pranayama with respiration.

> The yogi should apply a comfortable asana, then slowly draw in (samakrshya) wind (pavan, a synonym of vayu) by the southern (daksha; can also mean earth, wise, dexterous) nadi. (HYP 2, 48)

'Samakrshya pavan' is commonly translated as 'draw in air' or 'breathe in'. It is not air but 'parvan', a synonym of vayu, that is drawn in, which happens during the exhalation. 'Daksha nadi' is translated commonly as 'right nostril', but it is the southern or earthy nadi. Taking into account the name of the practice 'penetration of the sun', I see reason to define the 'dakha nadi' as the surya, the navel centre. After 'parvan' is drawn in *by* 'daksha nadi' (dakshanadya, instrumentalis), there follows a kumbhaka, which happens after the exhalation, then 'slowly pavan should be rechayet (expanded) into the (savya nadi) southern/right nadi' (HYP 2, 49). The vayu then is expanded into the southern or right side of the pranic body.

Ujjayi is described in the HYP:

> Having drawn the wind (pavana) slowly from the two nadis (nadibhyam) by controlling the head, hold it between the throat and the heart producing a sound. (HYP 2, 51)

Ujjayi is the well-known and much-used sonorous breath. I understand the controlling of the head to mean a long straight neck and the chin lowered for the throat contraction that produces the sound. The vayu moves up and down on the right and left side of the pranic body (both nadis), the expanding and reversing of the vayu, with the focus on the area between throat and heart: 'it can be performed in all conditions of life, even while walking or sitting' (HYP 2, 53).

The next two kumbhakas do not work on the pranic body, but on the physical. **Sitkari** (sound of breath) is a practice which uses words like 'mouth', 'nose' and 'drawing in of air'. The vocabulary used for sitkari is very different from the vocabulary used for pranayama (HYP 2, 54). There is no 'puraka' or 'rechaka', but 'vijrmbha', meaning 'open mouth or yawning'. And this open mouth activity does not take place in 'nadis', but in 'vaktra' (mouth, jaw) and in 'ghrana' (nose). Air is drawn down the breathing tubes, having a cooling result. There does not seem to be any relation to pranayama.

Sitali is the same practice as sitkari with the tongue poking out of the mouth and rolled. This also is a practice with no apparent relation to pranayama. It is done for cooling, which is a very useful practice in a hot country.

Bhastrika (little bag) in this context means bellows. Puraka, the drawing in of marut, is performed again and again in a powerful way like the bellows of a blacksmith. The bellows-like movement of marut is also done during the inhalation; bellows blow the air out to invigorate the fire. The abdominal wall moves fast inwards and outwards. This is a powerful practice leading to an awakening of kundalini (HYP 2, 66) and it breaks through the granthis, internal knots created by attachments (HYP 23, 67). Bhastrika is a practice that increases the duration of the kumbhaka and as such is a useful practice to facilitate pranayama.

Brahmari (bee) is humming, making sounds like a bee. The HYP does not give us many instructions, but just says that brahmari causes bliss (ananda). Bhramari has a calming effect and elongates the vayu reverse and the exhalation, thus reducing the impurities that block the vayu reverse. It is a beautiful practice for students who find it difficult to let breath just flow on its own, and most practitioners will be astonished how long the exhalation becomes when humming. Many students find focusing on the breath difficult at first and become confused about breathing. Brahmari is a wonderful practice for them to become more comfortable with letting breath happen.

Murcha (faint, not active, mentally still). After puraka, reversing of the vayu, close the throat with a jalandhara bandha (throat lock) and hold it. This practice uses the help of a bandha to remain in the state of kumbhaka, the state of mental stillness, and is therefore related to pranayama.

Plavini (spreading) is the practice of filling the belly with air to be able to float in water. It is a practice which has no relation to pranayama – it is a little odd, but may be useful.

Some of those kumbhakas are classified as pranayama in modern Yoga, but they are not: pranayama is nothing other than the natural movement of the vayu in the rhythm of the breath – expand, reverse and remain. No specific technique is needed for pranayama. Some of the kumbhakas, however, may be very helpful in encouraging the pranayama process and the removal of the impurities (malakulsa): the process that occurs in pranamaya kosha.

Practical: purifying the nadis

Apply a half or, if comfortable, a full lotus seat. Place the right foot on to the left thigh and ease the knee down to the floor. Use a blanket under the ankle bone if the thigh hurts. A block can be placed under the bent knee if it feels too intense. If possible, place the left foot under the already bent leg or even on the opposite thigh. The posture needs to be comfortable; if you strain, you will tense up.

Observe the vayu movement with emphasis on apana, the downwards movement. Send the expanding vayu from the mid-abdomen to the area of the right hip, and only the right hip. Pinpoint the main resistance without creating the image of tight hip muscles. Feel the restriction and know it is an impurity on a subtler level, something that clings, holds on. This restriction is not just blocking the way, but seems to have its own mind. The restrictions (mala) cling (kulasa) in the subtle body and come from the Ego part of mind – they are attachments. Allow the reverse of apana back to the mid-abdomen; allow it to loosen some of the impurities, the clinging and blocking, and bring them back into agni, your inner fire, to burn them. Visualize the reverse as a stream taking all unwanted debris along to carry it to its destination. Sharpen your focus, continue with the practice for a while and then stretch the legs out, sit in dandasana and observe. You should find that the right hip area is freed from some clinging elements and feels more expansive and open than the left.

You have not achieved the removal of blockages by stretching lots of muscles but by focus on pranayama.

The link between Prana and citta

The definition of Yoga as stated in the classical Yoga tradition (Raja Yoga), the Yoga Sutras of Patanjali, is:

Yogah citta vritti niorodha. (Patanjali 1, 2)

Yoga is the cessation of movements in the mind, citta.

There is no mention of the subtle body (pranamaya kosha), impurities, vayu and Prana, but the verse describes the same process.

Citta is a space in which mental activity takes place (manomaya kosha). The activities come in three forms. Manas, the filter, is the capacity that chooses from all sense perceptions a small number to enter conscious awareness. Buddhi, the intellect, connects the registered sense perceptions with each other, memorizes them and make sense of them. Ahankar, the Ego maker, creates an entity which relates the information to a 'me' and reacts with attachments.

Vritti is any activity, a movement, behaviour, occupation.

Nirodha means cessation.

The message of this verse is that citta needs to be stilled of any sense perceptions (manas), intellectual connections, memories (buddhi) and attachments (ahankar). How do Prana and pranayama relate to this?

Different Yoga traditions describe different pathways to the enlightened state – samadhi, unmani... The enlightened state is always the same. Traditions are like paths up a mountain; each path has a different starting point and the landscape looks different. Walking any path brings us to the peak, which is always the same. The Bhakti path of the Bhagavad Gita reaches the peak by surrendering the Ego to the Divine. The Karma path of the Bhagavad Gita reaches the path by detachment in action. The Jnana path of the Upanishads reaches the peak by realizing the Self. The Raja path of Patanjali reaches the peak by stilling the mind. The Hatha path reaches the peak by purifying the nadis, awakening kundalini and raising the pranic forces up sushumna.

When the Ego is surrendered to the Divine (Bhakti Yoga), actions can become detached (Karma Yoga). The cause of attachments is avidya, ignorance – not seeing that our destiny is the Self instead of the satisfaction of the Ego. Overcoming avidya leads to vidya, insight (Jnana Yoga). The result of overcoming attachments, the most obstinate movements in citta, is an open, empty mind space (Raja Yoga). The same attachments manifest themselves in the pranic level as mala kulasa, the clinging obstacles in the nadis. Pranayama is the detachment process that loosens the attachments in pranamaya kosha, leading to freedom and stillness in manomaya kosha. The methods of the different paths complement each other.

> When vata (wind) moves, citta (mind) moves, when vata is still, citta is. The Yogin obtains firmness, therefore vayu (wind) should cease. (HYP 2, 2)

The stilling of the mind will reduce the attachments and thus the impurities in the nadis. The practice of pranayama reduces the mala kulasa and thus leads to a still mind. The still mind causes the vayu movement to cease, and kevala kumbhaka occurs. No breath and no activity in the mind is the enlightened state.

Yoga practitioners know the experience of a still place after a complete 'exhalation', kumbhaka. We all experience stillness and a composed mental state when breath is absent.

Before I studied the Hatha verses in depth, I attempted to make sense of the ability to release with 'exhalation'. I taught my students that inhalation is a process of contracting all the breathing muscles and exhalation is the relaxation of the same muscles; the body relaxes with exhalation, not with inhalation. That is true in parts of the body where breathing muscles are located, but the effect of a complete Prana reverse and release can also be felt in the legs, feet, arms, head and neck, and hips and shoulders. The relaxation of the breathing muscles would also not explain the mental unburdening and the heightened sense of inner aliveness. The release with the 'exhalation' is not just a physical phenomenon: the pranic body purifies, attachments are let go, and the result is peace and stillness of mind.

The goal of pranayama

As long as there are malas, vayu movement continues. When the system is fully purified, the 'storm settles', the vayu becomes still and the 'sea calms'; there is just expanded Prana, kevala kumbhaka, and breathing has stopped.

This is the goal of pranayama and it is clearly stated in the above quoted verses HYP 2, 2-6. The words 'tato vayum nirodhayet' – therefore cease the vayu – form the end of verse 2 as well as verse 3, with identical wording.

If pranayama were a respiratory practice, then the goal would be an increase in lung capacity – more breath. Pranayama is not a respiratory practice, but Prana expansion. The further the Prana expansion proceeds, the less air flows up, to the extent that 'breathing' feels as if there is no more respiration, only pranayama. Kumbhaka occurs at first for a short moment – pauses between the breathing cycles – but it will become longer until breathing ceases. Before we are born, we do not breathe – life is maintained by Prana through the umbilical cord into our navel centre. When reaching kevala kumbhaka, we return to this state; we do not need to breathe any more, but live from Prana within.

Refrain

Pranayama is not respiration, but the expansion of Prana. Pranayama is a process not in the physical body but in the pranic body. Prana is not air or breath, but life that enters each embryo and settles in the navel centre; death occurs when Prana, life, leaves.

Pranayama, the expansion of Prana, is a threefold process: (1) the expanding of Prana from its origin in the navel centre outwards; (2) the reversing of Prana back to the navel centre; and (3) the containing of Prana in the navel centre. The threefold process is called vayu, and it happens in the rhythm of the breath, but it is not breath, and it moves in the opposite direction to respiration. Vayu does not move through air tubes but through nadis. The nadis are full of impurities, and pranayama is the purification process. Once the nadis are purified, the vayu stops moving and breath ceases. Prana then remains for prolonged periods in the navel centre where it creates heat, which awakens a dormant pranic force sitting in the base chakra, kundalini. Kundalini rises in the innermost, spiritual nadi, sushumna; when it reaches the top, sahasrara, an enlightened state occurs.

Practical: from sahita to kevala

Prepare yourself for pranayama. Sit upright and bring your awareness to your navel centre, connecting to the vayu movement.

> Practise abdominal kapalabhati for a minute or two (as described in the section 'Kabalabhati' under 'Common techniques used to facilitate pranayama' earlier in this chapter), then witness the pranic movement. Let the expansion continue; it can feel as if it could go on for ever without breathing any more air into the lungs. Let this expansion be followed by a reverse of the vayu, which can also seem to last forever, without air leaving the lungs. Surrender the reversing vayu to the deeper inner space, away from the busyness of the outer world, thought and attachment. If thought or ambitions continue, then you will not be able to stay in that still space.
>
> With practice, you will experience sahitha kumbhaka, the pause after the exhalation, which is incomplete – just a pause that will be followed by a vayu expansion. With more practice, the kumbhaka becomes longer and can eventually transform into a prolonged kevala kumbhaka. Sense the stillness in kumbhaka – the absence of thought, the absence of attachments, just being, here and now, nothing more.

In kumbhaka, the vayu movement is still (nirodha). The power of kumbhaka directly affects the dormant form of Prana, kundalini, at the base chakra, muladhara; it awakens and it rises up in an inner pranic dimension, sushumna.

When kundalini reaches the crown, sahasrahra, the practitioner has reached an enlightened state, samadhi.

The goal of pranayama is the cessation of breath, the stillness of vayu, the state of kevala kumbhaka, the awakening of kundalini and the gradual rise of kundalini up sushumna.

> Through kumbhaka, kundalini awakes, through kundalini awakening, sushumna becomes unblocked and perfection in Hatha arises. (HYP 2, 75)

What is kundalini?

The Sanskrit 'kundala' means 'coil, ring, snake'. Kundalini is the feminine form. The kundalini power was always associated with female Divinities in Indian history. It is one of the six expressions of individual Prana, the only one residing not in manipura, but in muladhara.

Kundalini is a major topic in Tantra and Hatha Yoga, but knowledge of the dormant power and the necessity to awaken it was present in India throughout its whole history and also in other cultures. The Orthodox Christian icon art depicts the experience of a kundalini rising to the crown of the head with a halo. The Mayans knew the high dormant force within and called it 'hurikan'.

The phenomenon of kundalini was already known in the Rig Veda. The Taittiriya Upanishad gives a list of practices and life principles for the householder in Part I, 9–10, and names 'raise kundalini' as one of them; that was long before the Hatha times. Georg Feuerstein said that kundalini was 'encountered by mystics throughout the ages' (Feuerstein 1990).

The understanding of kundalini was refined in Tantra and Hatha times and the phenomenon was often referred to with other names: 'Kutilangi, Kundalini, Bhujangini, Sakti, Isvari, Kundali and Arundhati are all synonymous words' (HYP 3,104).

Swami Satyananda Saraswati defines kundalini as follows: 'Kundalini is the name of a sleeping dormant potential force in the human organism and it is situated at the root of the spinal column' (Swami Satyananda Saraswati 1996b, p.5).

Other definitions are:

- 'Kundalini or serpent power is an energy latent in the body said to be coiled at the base of the spine' (Hewitt 1991, p.460).
- 'the divine cosmic force in our bodies' (Iyengar 1991, p.439).
- a 'mysterious psychospiritual force' (Feuerstein 1990).
- 'The great goddess Kundalini, the energy of Self, atma-shakti sleeps in muladhara' (GS 3, 12).

The above quotations describe a power in dormant form within the human system, a divine power. Yoga compositions speak about the possibility and necessity of awakening this power to fulfil human destiny. The way to awaken it is correct Yoga practice.

Kundalini is like nuclear energy. Any minute, harmless-looking nucleus of every atom can, when it is known how, be opened to release immense energy. This energy can be used for creative or destructive purposes. Kundalini is that power within individual beings.

Kundalini is the supreme power. (HYP 3, 51)

Can life remain alive in dormant form, invisible, inactive for a long time? It can, and we know that phenomenon very well. We can keep seeds in packets for years in a cupboard – brown, dead-looking little bits. There is no life to be seen when we open one up, but if we add water, life sprouts and a plant grows with the potential to grow many more seeds and many more plants. In the same way, having been dormant for lifetimes, kundalini can awaken when the vayu reverse becomes complete, through correct Yoga practice. Because this invisible, dormant life remains a mystery that cannot be comprehended, Kundalini was therefore linked to the Divine. It is the concentrated form of Shakti; the Goraksha Paddhati, the Hatha Yoga Pradipika and other compositions call it 'the Great Goddess'.

Old and modern sources define kundalini as an immense source of dormant energy; psychic healers can see it.

Krishnamacharya and his followers nevertheless have a different take: that kundalini is not a power, but a blockage, a knot, like a granthi, sitting at the opening of sushumna and not letting Prana pass. Yoga practices would not awaken it, but only remove the blockage so that Prana can enter sushumna. All evidence speaks against this theory. It could be one of Krishnamacharya's attempts to demystify Yoga and make it digestible for Western thinking.

Where is kundalini located?

Krishnamacharya got his idea from statements like 'Kundalini sleeps covering the entrance of the region of Brahman' (sushumna) (HYP 3, 106). Kundalini sits at the opening of sushumna, which is within muladhara chakra, and yes, it prevents Prana rising up into the spiritual channel, but it is far more than a blockage that needs removing. It is a goddess, a dormant power, an immense power, which, when awakened and rising up sushumna, can cause enlightened experiences and insight.

Kundalini is depicted as a snake with three and a half coils – the Goraksha Paddhati speaks about eight coils, (I, 47). The symbol of a snake stands for a mysterious power. The three coils symbolize the three gunas; the half is an Indian way of stating, 'whatever cannot be expressed'.

Is Kundalini different from Prana?

The list of synonyms in HYP 3, 104 (see above) shows that kundalini and shakti are considered to be the same. Feuerstein calls kundalini the 'individualised form of shakti' (Feuerstein 1990).

Swami Satyananda Saraswati says that the energy known as prana shakti, the universal life force in the Indian mythology, is called kundalini in Tantra (Swami Satyananda Saraswati 1996b, p.6). Kundalini is Prana in a very highly concentrated form.

When Kundalini awakens, it rises upward into sushumna, which is a deeper spiritual dimension within the network of nadis. Kundalini-Prana entering brings life into the deeper spiritual dimensions, and gives rise to insight of these planes, which are otherwise closed to perception.

What happens when kundalini awakens?

In normal circumstances, kundalini awakens very, very slowly, over years, decades or even lifetimes. On rare occasions, sudden awakenings are reported. 'Kundalini Yoga' aims for fast awakenings. One needs to be far enough evolved on the path of human development to channel this strong force safely. The pot needs to be strong to contain the content. Forced awakening can cause serious problems. Krishna Gopi (1993) described in his autobiography a sudden kundalini awakening. He was not ready for it and suffered for 20 years from disturbed mental and physical health until he built up the strength to house the awakened power.

In the context of pranayama, each complete reverse of the vayu followed by kumbhaka disturbs kundalini and causes some rising. A lightness and awareness from the 'base of the spine' upwards is experienced in a slight and slow manner.

A highly awakened kundalini gives significant power, which can be used for creative or destructive purposes – kundalini is neutral. When not morally advanced, kundalini can take the form of Kali energy (the dark destructive goddess); when morally advanced, it takes the form of Durga energy (the benign, beautiful goddess). The Kali kundalini can cause serious damage and powerful destruction. According to Swami Satyananda Saraswati, a person who is about to commit murder has an awakened Kali kundalini. 'Successful' destructors, like Hitler, could be seen to have an active kundalini.

A person experiencing kundalini rising as Durga energy develops vidya and jnana, achieves understanding of the ways and the purpose of the universe and the individual Self, and gains siddhis, special powers. Spiritual knowledge does not arise with a complete dormant kundalini. Einstein did not have a bigger brain than other scientists; he had an awakened kundalini. Creativity is also a sign of Durga awakening, having access to planes of higher beauty; Mozart had an active kundalini. Some awakened people are powerful role models and leaders like Mahatma Gandhi, Mother Teresa and Amma. The ability to reach and enthuse others, which we call charisma, without any explanation of what that might be, is an active kundalini. A fully rising kundalini leads to the enlightened state.

The process of kundalini rising is described in the Hatha writings:

- 'Kundalini is drawn into sushumna and lifts' (HYP 3, 117).
- 'the awakened kundalini it moves upwards through sushumna' (Feuerstein 2001, p.405, quoting the Goraksha Paddhati).

The aim of kundalini is the crown of the head, shahsrara. When it reaches this place, 'new consciousness dawns' (Swami Satyananda Sarswati 1996b, p.6).

Do only special people have an awakened kundalini?

A fully awakened kundalini can indeed only be found in very special, enlightened people. They have extinguished the Ego and are fully detached, compassionate and in possession of special skills, siddhis. Partially awakened kundalini is very common.

Krishna Gopi names as a sign of a rising kundalini the desire to transform one's life, and that is common. People who realize that life has a meaningful purpose, who try to find their path of self-development and want to become better people, are driven by kundalini power. There are others who don't see the necessity of inward progression. They describe 'seekers' as people with problems; they have a dormant kundalini. There is no way to explain to a person with a dormant kundalini the necessity of a spiritual path. Leave them be and focus on your own journey.

The further along we move on a spiritual path, the more kundalini will awaken. According to the Indian belief system, we will not lose an awakening with death. When reincarnating, we start on the level we left.

We are all at different stages of evolution, and in some of us kundalini may have already reached swadhisthana, manipura or anahata chakra. (Swami Satyananda Saraswati 1996b, p.6)

How to awaken kundalini: the evidence in the Hatha compositions

There is only one way to awaken kundalini, and that is, as described above, the cessation of breath, kumbhaka. There are nevertheless many ways that lead to kumbhaka. Not just pranayama, but meditation also leads to kumbhaka. People who practise meditation regularly report that they sometimes breathe very little. When in awe, the state of jnana, the breath stops. The Hatha verses show us that breath ceases when the impurities, mala kulasa, are gone, when attachments are overcome. The path of Bhakti Yoga surrenders the Ego to the Divine and the breath will cease, at least temporarily. Karma Yoga cultivates detached actions, Jnana Yoga removes avidya, ignorance, and Raja Yoga nips attachments in the bud by preventing them from growing in the mind space. All these methods lead to the cessation of breath.

Pranayama, the purification of the nadis, leads to the ceasing of breath and awakening of kundalini.

> Kumbhaka awakes kundalini; through arousing kundalini, sushumna becomes freed and siddhi (perfection) in Hatha Yoga arises. (HYP 2, 75)

Pranayama leads to kumbhaka, and kumbhaka leads to the awakening of kundalini; once kundalini is awakened, other practices can aid in the rise. Mudras and bandhas fulfil this purpose:

- 'Jalandhara bandha lifts the pranic force up in sushumna' (HYP 3, 11).
- Asana help to raise kundalini – those specifically mentioned are ardha matsyendrasana (1, 27) and padmasana (1, 48).

I remember sitting in a British Wheel of Yoga meeting a few years ago, when someone said that kundalini rising is not something we work with, and none of us would have any experience of it. Statements like this have two origins. First, most people have read stories of sudden, amazing kundalini awakenings and think that kundalini awakening happens only in this way. Second, the old instructions of the HYP and other compositions are not followed; they are replaced by modern anatomical explanations which do not lead the practitioner's awareness to perceive subtle changes like kundalini.

I had no sudden kundalini rising, but I know very well what kundalini feels like and know how to work with it, and so do my students. It is possible to instruct even beginners in a way that they feel a rising aliveness and power.

Practical: learning to sense kundalini

With some understanding of the process of pranayama and help from practices that facilitate kumbhaka, you can learn to use the initially short phase of kumbhaka in all your Yoga practice.

Stand in tadasana and expand the vayu from the navel centre; allow an unrestricted reverse and enter kumbhaka. In kumbhaka, drop the roots of the big toes and the inner heels; your knees will roll outwards slightly, the inner arches will lift, and you will have the sensation of the sacrum becoming upright. Apply shambhavi mudra (turn your eyes up to the point between your eyebrows) and kechari mudra (roll the tongue back and point the tip of the tongue to ajna chakra). Both mudras help to rise from the ajna chakra region upwards. The drawing from the feet down and rising with the mudras up opens the space along sushumna. Now lower into uttanasana (standing forward bend) in kumbhaka by lifting the 'sitting bone' area away from the dropping roots of the big toes; the head and chest will lower. Space will open up, and you might assume that you feel the sacrum. You do not feel the sacrum, because we cannot feel bones; what you feel is a rising aliveness, kundalini.

The same process can be applied in pashimottanasana (sitting forward bend) as long as the spine is not rounded, the pelvis is tilted, the sitting bones move backwards, the roots of the big toes move away from the body and both mudras are applied. In kumbhaka, you can feel an awareness moving up in the sacrum area.

You can sit in baddha konasana (soles joined), link into pranayama and shift the knees outwards during kumbhaka to open the sacrum area, where a similar aliveness can be felt.

When more confident with the lower sushumna awareness, find asana that enable you to open higher parts.

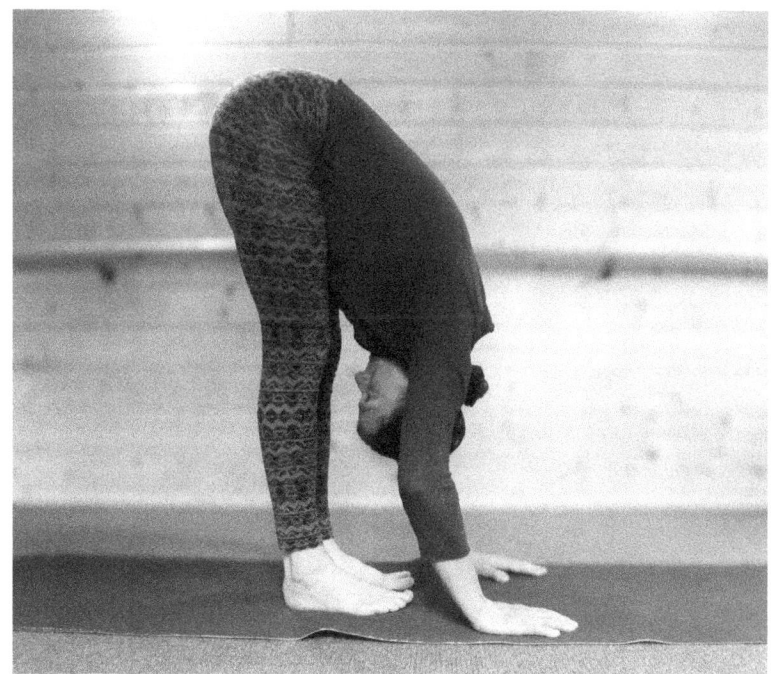

Figure 4.2 *Uttanasana*

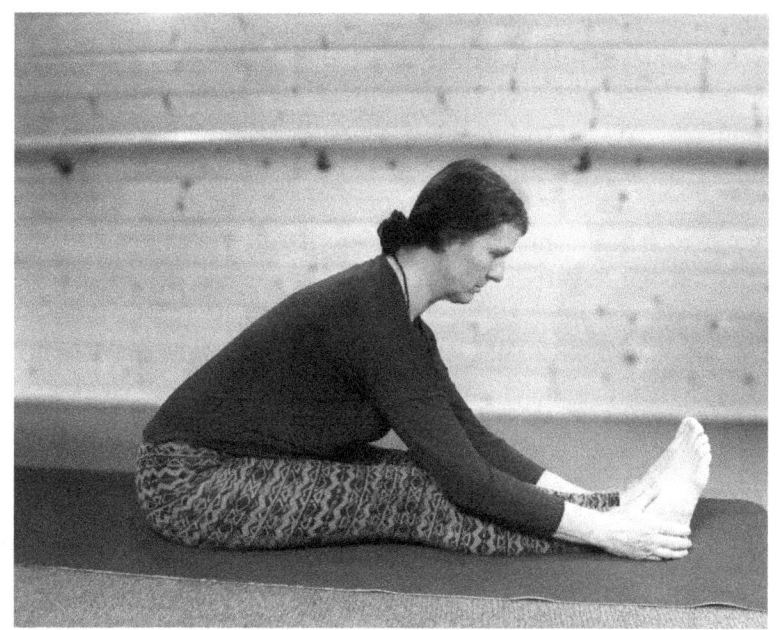

Figure 4.3 *Pashimottanasana*

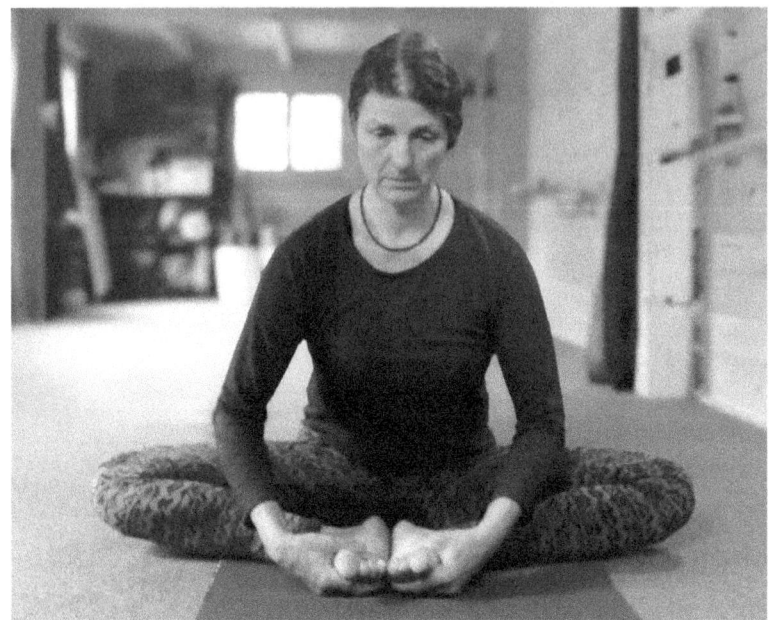

Figure 4.4 *Baddha konasana*

Pranayama in non-Hatha traditions

The Vedas do not instruct pranayama, The concept of Prana is known in the old hymns, but practice in the early Vedic period was limited to chanting and rituals. Later in the era of the Upanishads, when seekers settled in solitude in forests or mountains, it was meditation that was practised. The Prashna Upanishad describes the vayu, in answer to the question of a seeker:

> Master, from what source does this prana come? How does he enter the body, how live after dividing himself into five? (Easwaran 1988, Prashna Upanishad, Question III, 1)

The master does not instruct pranayama, but explains the function of the vayu, so that the seekers can see it in meditation, a Jnana Yoga approach.

The Bhagavad Gita gives plenty of Bhakti (dedication to the Divine) and Karma Yoga (detached action) instructions. Prana is only instructed once in the context of meditation, in chapter 5: 'pranapanau samau krtva', making prana and apana movement the same (Bhagavad Gita 5, 27).

Prana and apana are not explained, and were therefore obviously known by people chanting and listening to the Bhagavad Gita. These three words are translated as 'steady the breathing' (Feuerstein 2014) or 'equalize the in and the out breaths' (Sri Swami Satchidananda 1988) or 'making the in-breath and the out-breath more [even]' (Feuerstein 2014). Making prana and apana the same is not equalizing the inhalation and exhalation, but allowing the vayu movement to reach equally up and down; there is no mention of the duration of the phases. If apana has more emphasis, a tamasic (dull, lazy) slumping can occur; the emphasis on prana can result in rajastic (active, with intent) ambition. These three words reveal the experience of pranayama by the verse composers.

In the Sutra compositions between 500 and 300 BCE we do find instructions on pranayama. The Patanjali Yoga Sutras dedicate four verses (2, 49–52) to pranayama in the description of the eight limbs; pranayama is the third limb of Yoga. Considering the density of sutras, four verses is a complex instruction.

Pranayama as described in Patanjali 2, 49–52

Verse 2, 49 announces pranayama, which is then defined in the next verse:

> *Bahya abhyantara sthambha vritti desha kala samkhyabhih paridhrshto dirghasuksham.* (Patanjali 2, 50)

> Outwards, inwards and suspended are the movements that need to be learned in the right place, time and number and they are long or short.

Bahya = outwards; abhyantara = thoroughly inwards; sthambha = stationary, suspended; vritti = movement; desha = place; kala = time; samkhyabhih = by number; paridhrshto = seen, learned; dirgha = long; suksham = short.

Two familiar words appear here, which we do not find in the Hatha pranayama instructions: **bahya** (outwards) and **abhyantara** (thoroughly inwards). Those two words are not connected to kumbhaka, but describe the Prana expansion outwards and backwards; the two words do not appear in association with 'kumbhaka'. 'Bahya' is an adjective meaning external. Patanjali uses this word in 2, 49. The root of the word is 'bah' and can also form the preposition 'bahih', outside. When this preposition is followed by a word beginning with a soft consonant such as 'g', the second 'h' changes to 'r', as in 'bahirgrama', the outhouse. The change from 'h' to 'r' does not happen when followed by a hard consonant like 'k'. When describing an outside kumbhaka, it would be 'bahih kumbhaka' and not 'bahir kumbhaka', which is grammatically incorrect. Those Western Yogis who coined the term 'bahir kumbhaka' have obviously not found it in the Sanskrit tradition, but have made it up and got it wrong.

When we learned the four phases of breath – puraka, antara kumbhaka, rechaka and bahir kumbhaka – in my Yoga teacher training, I asked my tutor why Patanjali speaks about three phases if there are actually four. The answer was that both retentions count as one phase. This does not make sense: one is after the inhalation and the other after the exhalation – how could they be counted as one? In my study of Yoga compositions, I have never come across four stages of pranayama, nor have I seen the words bahya or antara linked with the term kumbhaka.

There are three phases, not four. Bahya is not describing a pause but an outward movement; not the outward movement of air, exhalation, but the outward movement of the pranic fields from the origin of all nadis, the navel centre, which happens during the inhalation. Antara is not describing a pause but an inward movement; not an inward movement of air, inhalation, but an inward movement of the pranic fields from the origin of all nadis, the navel centre, which happens during the exhalation. Sthamba is Patanjali's term for kumbhaka, which happens after the pranic reverse, exhalation.

Patanjali does not speak about vayus and pranic fields at this point; he mentions vayus in chapter 3. This verse, Patanjali 2, 50, is in perfect agreement with HYP 2, 71 formulated 1500 years later, which we aleady analysed:

Pranayama is said to have three elements, rechaka (expand out) puraka (fill in), and kumbhaka (literally pot, here referring to the pause after the exhalation). (HYP 2,71)

Using these three elements bahya, antara and stambha, one should learn to bring them in the right place, timing and number. Patanjali does not mention a place from where these movements should take place. I assume it is the navel centre, kanda, the origin of all nadis – this is where the movement is felt. The later Hatha tradition does name the place as surya chakra. Time and number refer to the duration of each phase and how often this threefold process is to be repeated. Detailed instruction on time and number is not given. Bearing in mind that these verses are sutras – maximum information in minimum number of words – there is lot of information. A sutra is a mnemonic to be kept in mind by regular chanting, to remind the practitioner of the master's instructions.

Practical: pranayama à la Patanjali

Practise pranayama in its three phases: bahya (outward moving), antara (inward moving) and stambha (stationary). Those three phases are to be carried out in the right place, time and number.

This practice is not complicated, but in its simplicity it is very challenging. Just sit and breathe, do not achieve breath – do not even breathe; the breath occurs on its own, and all you have to do is stop doing. The practice is the witnessing of a movement from the **place** (desha) where the whole movement originates from. Most of the time, our centre of awareness sits in the head; now bring it into the belly. You want to be in the right starting place. Witness the three phases from that place; expand out, reverse back and remain. Stay in the mid-abdomen as the expansion outwards occurs; do not move along to the places the pranic forces go. Imagine you sit in the mid-abdomen, your home, and from there shines life and light outwards; you look out, but do not go along with it – you stay at home.

This movement has a **time** duration; don't manipulate it – it will slow down. All three phases will elongate, but at the same time the amount of air breathed will decrease. The sthamba in particular will prolong when the need to do the breath is gone and you are not ahead of yourself, already in the next phase.

You breathe 24 hours a day. If the breath stays unaware and thus manipulated by mind, attachments, rush, stress and fear, then spending five minutes of those 24 hours on pranayama is not much help. The awareness in this process and the detaching from the need to do it has to take up more and more of our time, so that the **number** will increase. You have to focus on other things during the day, but you can allow the pranic movement to become an underlying foundation of your life and try to find moments – gaps in daily life – when you can return with full attention to it.

The next verse:

Bahyabhyantara vishayakshepi caturthah. (Patanjali 2, 51)

Transcended the sphere of bahir and antara, a fourth (state) reached.

Bahya = outwards; abhyantara = thoroughly inwards; vishaya = domain, sphere, matter; akshepi = transcend, overcome; caturthah = the fourth.

The pranic expansion outward (bahya) and inward (antara) transcended means the vayu is no longer moving; it is still. Not temporarily – that would be stambha, or sahitha kumbhaka in Hatha terms – but for a prolonged time. As the vayu is a movement sharing the same rhythm as the respiration, not just the vayu movement but also the respiration stops. In the Patanjali Sutras, this fourth state is not given a name; the later Hatha tradition calls this phenomenon 'kevala kumbhaka'. This stillness is not a longer pause, but freedom from all the movement that distorts the clear sight of the inner Self.

Tatah kshiyate prakasha avaranam. (Patanjali 2, 52)

As a result, the covering over the inner light wanes.

Tatah = after that; kshiyate = wane, perish, waste away; prakasha = inner light; avaranam = cover.

The suspended breath removes the covering of an inner luminosity. Prakasha is a term which is used in Indian philosophy to describe the light making the inner conscious Self (Atman, Purusha) apparent. Prakasha is 'one of the two aspects of Paramashiva, the Ultimate Reality. It is the principle of self-revelation which illuminates everything; consciousness; the principle by which everything else is known' (Grimes 1996).

When prakasha is fully uncovered through the practice of pranayama, then Self-realization can be reached.

Practical: the uncovering of the inner light

Return to your pranayama practice as described above. Do not try to control the three phases; just focus and 'look' at the pause, kumbhaka. Practise from kumbhaka to kumbhaka; dwell in this space. You are not ready to remain there for good; attachments keep the movements going, but reach for the kumbhaka. This is your home. If you lead a busy life, leaving home in the morning and coming back in the evening, the time will come when you retire and stay at home.

When you have become more settled and comfortable in the kumbhaka, visualize that entering kumbhaka is like entering a temple or a cathedral. At first it seems dark, but move into the centre of the place, and there is a transparent dome in middle of the ceiling and light is reaching down to you. When this image works, then let go of it; just be in your kumbhaka and realize your inner lightness intensifying. 'Then the cover over the inner light wanes' (Patanjali 2, 52).

Although the Patanjali composition is 1500 years earlier than Hatha, we find the same principles. The same experience has been passed on for many generations.

Pranayama in Patanjali is, as in the Hatha tradition, not a breathing practice with the aim of increasing lung capacity or improving respiratory health. Pranayama is not the so-called 'complete Yoga breath', a completion of breath in all three respiratory areas – diaphragmatic, thoracic and clavicular. Pranayama is not a collection of specific techniques. Pranayama is a threefold movement of outwards, inwards and stationary. The practice of pranayama leads to the cessation of the breathing movement, where the covering over the inner light disappears.

There is nevertheless another state that can occur when the exhalation is no longer followed by an inhalation; that is called death. In death, the vayu leaves the body, and all life goes. In the still phases of pranayama, the life force enters the inner middle, sushumna, to be contained, and it brings life to dimensions within us which were dormant before. No one has ever died from the correct practice of pranayama. Pranayama is entirely different from death; the need for breath is overcome. There is no danger in pranayama, only peace and stillness; breath will return when the stillness is broken by mind activities and life continues. No one has ever come to harm by ceasing to breathe in pranayama, but people have damaged their health by holding their breath after an inhalation. Medical science does not believe that a state of breath cessation can be survived, as most of the observation subjects have been non-enlightened non-yogis.

Chapter 5

BANDHAS

> **Refrain**
> Pranayama is not respiration, but the expansion of Prana. Pranayama is a process not in the physical body but in the pranic body. Prana is not air or breath, but life that enters each embryo and settles in the navel centre; death occurs when Prana, life, leaves.
> Pranayama, the expansion of Prana, is a threefold process: (1) the expanding of Prana from its origin in the navel centre outwards; (2) the reversing of Prana back to the navel centre; and (3) the containing of Prana in the navel centre. The threefold process is called vayu, and it happens in the rhythm of the breath, but it is not breath, and it moves in the opposite direction to respiration. Vayu does not move through air tubes but through nadis. The nadis are full of impurities, and pranayama is the purification process. Once the nadis are purified, the vayu stops moving and breath ceases. Prana then remains for prolonged periods in the navel centre where it creates heat, which awakens a dormant pranic force sitting in the base chakra, kundalini. Kundalini rises in the innermost, spiritual nadi, sushumna; when it reaches the top, sahasrara, an enlightened state occurs.

Kumbhaka, the cessation of the vayu and awakening of kundalini, is initially not long enough to raise kundalini all the way up to sahasrara. The rising of kundalini is also inhibited by obstructions. Not only is the outer pranic body full of impurities (malas), but the inner pranic body, sushumna, has its own obstructions, 'granthis' (knots).

Nature has equipped us with inner mechanisms that can become active in kumbhaka to assist kundalini to rise. These inner mechanisms ensure a longer kumbhaka and shift through the granthis to loosen them. The mechanisms are called bandhas, which are in a way the extension of pranayama. Bandhas are, like pranayama, not processes within the anatomical body. When the practitioner is advanced enough in pranayama to reach a prolonged kumbhaka, then bandhas take over: they are advanced practices: 'Bandhas are very advanced and complex practices, even difficult to attain by the Maruts (divinities)' (GS 3, 5).

All these Sanskrit phenomena would sound very daunting if we were merely scholars. But we are also practitioners and have followed the Yogis' instructions and come to experiences that cannot be expressed in language. When the old Hatha Yogis formulated their wisdom, they did not want to create a theory or a model; rather, they experienced inner processes, found ways of influencing the inner processes and tried to find words to express the experience. All these words are only of use when we focus inwards and follow the directions of the Yogis to find the experience. Once were are in the experience, it does not matter at all whether we use their terminology or any other or none.

In modern Yoga, bandhas have been associated with core strength and muscular contractions, and students are instructed to squeeze and pull up. But the bandhas are neither locatable in the physical body nor muscular contractions. Bandhas move Prana, and *Prana is not moved by muscles, but by vayu*.

Yoga teachers with a good understanding know that bandhas are more complex events than contracting muscles. The Ashtanga Guru David Swenson, whose asana teaching is physically very demanding, acknowledges this fact:

> Bandhas are a series of internal energy gates within the subtle body which assist in the regulation of the pranic flow. (Swenson 1999, p.9)

Bandhas are not instructed as muscular contractions in the Hatha verses, nor are they done for physical benefits.

> The bandhakas, energy locks, of jalandhara, oddyana, and mula, have to be practised respectively, in the throat, stomach, and the base of the anus. If one knows and practises these three energy locks well, how can the cruel noose of time bind one. When the energy locks of oddyana, jalandhara, and mula awaken the coiled-up serpent-woman, kundalini,

then, the carrier of smell, air (wind) moves downwards towards the sushumna nadi, and gives up its going out and coming in (moves without coming and going, that is: no more vayu movement, the breath has ceased). (Yogataravali Sutras 5, 6)

This verse from the Yogataravali sums up the purpose of bandhas.

- Not bound by nose of time, free from time and mortality, no fear of death: attachments cause impurities (malas and granthis) in the pranic body, such as clinging to physical life, which ceases with the purification of that subtle plane. The rising kundalini assisted by the bandhas triggers higher states of consciousness and the immortal Self is realized. Fear of death will eventually be conquered. Many old verses state that bandhas conquer death. All Yoginis who have perfected the practice of bandhas have died, but by having become aware of the immortal Self, death is not death as in annihilation, but a mere transformation.
- Bandhas work on the pranic body: sushumna is opened and kundalini awakened.
- Bandhas become active in kumbhaka, in the state of no breath (the wind gives up its coming and going): they elongate the kumbhaka and enable the practitioner to remain longer in the state without breath.

The Sanskrit word 'bandha' has several meanings, from 'pack, bundle' to 'fastening, tie, bond'. In most modern Yoga books, it is translated as 'lock'. 'Locking' should not be understood as 'locking in' and 'holding back', but rather like the lock in a canal, channelling the water in the right direction, opening up for flow. Bandhas are opening and acceleration processes.

The old Yoga tradition classified bandhas as mudras (HYP chapter 3; GS chapter 4). Modern Yoga has given them their own category. There is a difference: mudras create pranic connections in the whole of the pranic body, whereas bandhas open dormant areas and actively move Prana onwards in sushumna only. Three main bandhas are:

- **mula bandha** (the root bandha): the mechanism lifting kundalini from the base chakra (muladhara) upwards

- **uddiyana bandha** (the flying up bandha): the lifting of kundalini from manipura upwards
- **jalandhara bandha** (the watergate bandha): the lifting of kundalini from the throat chakra (vishuddhi) upwards.

Maha bandha (the great bandha) is a combination of the three. **Maha veda** (the great knowledge) intensifies maha bandha by lifting the body in padmasana off the floor, with the aid of the bandhas.

Some new schools in Western Yoga have introduced pada bandha (foot bandha) and hasta bandha (hand bandha). Pada and hasta bandhas root the feet and hands when on the floor, as support for the three main bandhas. Pada and hasta bandha are not Indian traditions. They are not linked to sushumna and do not raise kundalini, and therefore they should not be associated with the bandhas, but they can be useful instructions.

The HYP regards uddiyana bandha as the best of the bandhas. Uddiyana bandha is the strongest, the most effective. The Bihar School of Yoga has emphasized the importance of mula bandha and considers it to be the 'master key' to unlocking the human potentials (Swami Buddhananda 1998a).

Mula bandha (MB)

The HYP and GS describe mula bandha as 'bending' (akuncan) of the 'lower pelvic area' (gudam) (HYP 3, 62). Gudam is a vague term referring to anything below the navel. MB instructions would have been given to a student by a master in a one-to-one situation. The instructions in the HYP are not meant to replace personal instruction and are therefore often not complete. Students who were instructed in bandhas would have been experienced in pranayama, would have had developed kumbhaka and would have known the experiences of a rising kundalini. 'Akuncayed gudam' is usually translated with 'contract the anus'. Anus is definitely the wrong term as it is the opening of the back passage, not the opening of sushumna. Contracting is a very active and muscular term and as such unsuitable. Akuncan, meaning bending, is better translated as straightening up, like straightening a bent pipe so that water can flow through. Bandhas are not done or achieved; they occur in focused practice, in postures such as simhasana: 'The three bandhas are made to come in action in this best asana' (HYP 1, 54).

It is not the ability to isolate and contract muscles that makes MB, but the advance of purification in the pranic body by pranayama, then bandhas; a sensation of lifting lightness in the inner core will be experienced.

> By this (reversing apana and prana) the sleeping kundalini is awakened by heat, it hisses and straightens like a snake hit by a stick. Then it enters Brahma nadi like a serpant enters a hole. Therefore the Yogis should always practise mula bahanda. (HYP 3, 67-68)

It is not the will of the practitioner that causes the activation of the bandhas, but the awakened power of kundalini. Instructing an inexperienced student in contracting the pelvic floor might tone their bodies but it does not lead to a yogic bandha experience.

Practical: mula bandha

Practise pranayama and allow the pranic reverse to come to a completion; a slight contraction of the abdominal wall can help. Allow the belly to be sucked in and keep the chin close to the chest without tilting the head forward. A fiery sparkling in the navel centre can be felt, marking the end of the reverse and the beginning of kumbhaka. Allow the area around your sitting bones to root down into the ground, but keep your bottom muscles and thighs relaxed. Let the inward sucking of the belly reach down to the base of your inner central axis to allow a rising from here to occur. It feels like an uncovering and awakening of muladhara chakra. The stiller the mind, the longer you will remain in this state. Muladhara chakra will cover up again at the end of the kumbhaka as the abdominal wall releases. The pranic forces expand outwards again from the navel centre for the next round. MB can eventually become an integrated part of your body rhythm and you will find a suggestion of MB naturally ending a 'breath cycle'.

MB raises the awakened kundalini from the first chakra, muladhara, to the third, manipura. Between those chakras within sushumna sits a major impurity, obstruction, a 'granthi' (knot). Granthis, like malas, are forms of attachments sitting in the nadis; the obstructions are called malas when situated in the ida/pingala network and granthis when situated in sushumna. When kundalini is awakened by kumbhaka, the lifting action of the bandhas can shift through the granthi and loosens it.

> Then (when kundalini rises) all lotuses (chakras) are loosened and also the granthis. (HYP 3, 2)

> The granthis prevent the free flow of prana along sushumna nadi and thus impede the awakening of the chakras and the rising kundalini. (Swami Satyananda Saraswati 1996a, p.407)

Granthis are mentioned in the Upanishads as blockages to our spiritual awakening. Chandogya Upanishad VII, 26.2 tells us that knowledge of the scriptures releases us from granthis. Katha Upanishad VI, 15 claims that the release of granthis leads to immortality. The Hatha tradition defines the granthis as attachments located in the pranic body, forming dark, impenetrable places. There are three main granthis named after the three main godheads, Brahma, Vishnu and Rudra (another name of Shiva). The location of the granthis differs slightly from tradition to tradition. Granthis are not in the physical body, which makes the description of a location imprecise and difficult. To simplify matters I will locate the lowest, **brahma granthi** (the knot of Brahma), in the space between muladhara and swatisthana (first and second chakra); the second, **vishnu granthi** (the knot of Vishnu), in the space between manipura and annahata (third and fourth chakra); and the highest, **rudra granthi** (the knot of Rudra), in the space between vishuddhi and ajna (fifth and sixth chakra).

Granthis prevent kundalini from rising upwards from the lower to the higher chakras. Independent from the Hatha knowledge, the modern therapy 'zero balancing' experiences dark spots in just those areas. They are called 'bottlenecks' and seen as situated in places where the skeletal system is closing in: in the lower pelvis, at the lower end of the ribcage and at the top of the neck where the skull closes in.

The Yoga Shikha Upanishad is said to use the analogy of a bamboo rod to describe granthis. The hollow rod is sushumna, and the partitions within the rod are the granthis; with the strength of the bandhas, these partitions can be pierced. Each of these 'granthis represent a particular state of consciousness or attachment, which acts as an obstacle on the path to higher awareness' (Swami Buddhananda 1998a, p.49).

Attachments to possessions create a dense, dark block in the pranic body in the lower pelvic area; this is brahma granthi. As long as this dense area is in place, we are not awakening beyond muladhara. MB can help to break attachment to possessions, but the practice needs to be accompanied by wilful detachment from possessions.

Possessions are not wrong per se, but the attachment to them can poison our inner being. Spiritual traditions of all times and places recommended poverty as the beginning of a spiritual journey. With higher self-control, ownership might no longer be harmful. However, many spiritual leaders from popes to Yogis were believed to be beyond attachment, but they became rich, attachments came back and they lost their way. When we are attached to what we own, or want to own, kundalini cannot rise up to swatisthana, which is the chakra that enables us to experience joy. As long as we are attached to possessions, we can't enjoy them.

Uddiyana bandha (UB)

Uddiyana means 'flying up'; the HYP speaks of Prana like a great bird flying up sushumna (HYP 3, 55). The instructions are minimal – just 'draw the belly in' – and breath in not mentioned. More refined instructions would have been given directly from the master.

UB is a powerful practice: it helps to complete the pranic reverse, elongates kumbhaka, increases the inner fire, rises kundalini another step higher and loosens vishnu granthi. Vishnu granthi is the dense, dark block created by attachments to people's opinion about us: peer pressure. It is a powerful obstacle; we are all much more dependent on other people's view of us than we are happy to admit. What we do, what we don't do, how we dress, how we speak, how we move, how we decorate our houses and where we go on holiday are all ruled by either wanting to fit in or wanting to stand out. Both come from the same attachment to others' views instead of what is right, what is wholesome, what is good for me, what makes me happy. A strong dependence on others' views shows in a low inner fire, the inability to allow UB bandha to occur. I see a lot of people with weak abdominal movement when they breathe, and they usually suffer pressure from outer norms. When they learn to increase the inner fire and increase the abdominal movement, then they gain more independence and power to stand for themselves.

Practical: uddiyana bandha

Practise UB on two levels, first the strong one, as a preliminary, and later a gentler UB combined with the other bandhas.

Here, I will give you very physical instructions. Respiration always accompanies pranayama and the strong physical practice will fire up the inner layers.

Care needs to be taken with the strong UB. It should not be done with any heart or eye conditions, pre- or antenatal or after recent abdominal surgery. It should also be avoided during heavy menstrual bleeding.

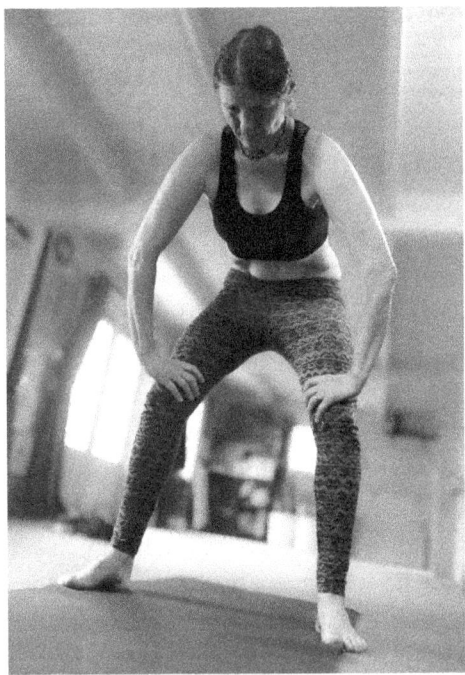

Figure 5.1 *Uddiyana bandha*

The best posture for UB is the 'skiing position'. Standing with the feet approximately 50 centimetres apart, bend forward with a rounded spine, hands on the knees. The tailbone is pointing downwards; keep your abdominal muscles loose for the exhalation to draw the belly in. Exhale completely with an open mouth and release the last air out of the lungs without being inhibited by a noisy breath. At the end of the exhalation, expel any remaining air out of the lungs. Let mula bandha and jalandhara bandha kick in. A vacuum in the lungs will lift the abdomen in and up; do not use strength of the abdominal muscles for the rise. On the pranic level, the rise comes from the power from manipura. When you get the hang of it, you might be astonished that the abdomen has become completely hollow. Remain here as long as comfortable, then slowly release the abdomen with the incoming breath. Have a few breaths in between and repeat up to three to six times, not more – the practice is very powerful. This practice will make your breath looser over time, your abdomen stronger and your pranayama more complete.

The second level is integrating UB into your pranayama. Each pranic reverse draws the abdominal wall in; the more complete reverse can feel like an active sucking in from the abdominal middle. The belly draws inwards and upwards having entered kumbhaka, and mula bandha will follow. This practice will be done in a seated asana to start with, but can be included more and more in all asana work.

Jalandhara bandha (JB)

There are several interpretations of the meaning of the word jalandhara: jal = throat; jaala = net; jalan = water; dhara = stream; adhara = gate (the 16 points which are locked by jalandhara). It doesn't seem to be clear which of those words formed the name originally.

HYP 3, 70 tells us to 'bend' (akuncan) the throat and bring the chin to the chest. Concerning the 'bending', see the section on MB above. The chin is placed down towards the chest by raising the highest neck vertebra, not by dropping the head. The cervical spine elongates and opens; it stays in alignment with the rest of the spine. The main purpose, as for all the bandhas, is lifting and raising of kundalini higher up sushumna. Neither the HYP nor the GS mention breath in the instructions. Jalandhara is performed in kumbhaka only. When kundalini has risen to the chest aided by the other bandhas, then the straightening and opening of the throat area can allow for kundalini to move on to ajna chakra.

Between vishuddhi and ajna is the location of the third granthi, rudra granthi. The Hatha Yogis have seen it as a dense, dark block of attachment to 'siddhis' (special powers). When kundalini has risen as far as vishuddhi, a lot of dormant potentials have activated and siddhis, higher abilities, will have occurred, such as a loose and strong body, high concentration levels, seeing events invisible to others, more insights occurring... The occurrence of siddhis happens in the detachment process; the practitioner feels less need for material things (brahma granthis is looser) and less urge to fit in with society (vishnu granthi is looser). The gain of special abilities nevertheless can give the Ego satisfaction and strengthen it again, which retrospectively causes rudra granthi to become dense and present itself as the next challenge. Siddhis are visible signs of progression and thus welcome, but care has to be taken. Stagnation occurs if the journey stops at this point. The Patanjali Yoga Sutras warn of attachment to siddhi (Patanjali 3, 38).

Being mindful and observant of the ways of the Ego and developing JB will help gradually to loosen the attachments to abilities and the need to succeed and excel. Kundalini will rise higher up to ajna and the awakened ajna will give the practitioner the ability to distinguish between Ego and Self.

Practical: jalandhara bandha

First, practise JB on its own. Adopt a straight seated position and lengthen the back of the neck, by raising from the last vertebra; do not drop the chin. JB is opening the inner throat and channelling the pranic forces upwards; the rise will help to loosen rudra granthi. The channelling upwards works best when trying to apply a swallow without finishing it. If that is difficult, take a sip of water into your mouth, swallow and observe how you do this. With the next sip of water start a swallow, but do not finish it. You will hold the water slightly higher up in the throat; when deciding not to swallow, the water comes down again. This is the action we are looking for. Now focus on pranayama. Let the pranic forces expand from the navel centre and allow them to reverse completely so that you can enter kumbhaka. Apply your half swallow. Sense a subtle rising. Release the bandha and allow the pranic forces to expand again.

Combining all three bandhas to a maha bandha, two ways are taught: either first mula, then uddiyana and then jalandhara bandha, or the other way round, jalandhara, uddiyana and mula. Logically, it might make sense to start with mula bandha. Swami Satyananda Saraswati nevertheless starts at jalandhara. Try it out. I feel the start with jalandhara helps me to abandon the image of pushing up and makes it feel like creating a vacuum, so that the rise happens of its own accord.

Continue with the practice and make it part of your daily experience. Experiment and learn through your own observation, and find more and more of the truth in the Hatha verses.

I was never taught swallowing to apply JB, nor did I receive any helpful instructions concerning the practice. Trying to come to terms with JB in my practice, I remembered a childhood event. I was keen on swimming and gained a number of swimming certificates. One task was swimming under water twice the length of the pool, 50 metres. We all found that difficult, and our swimming coach recommended swallowing a sip of water when we felt we could not carry on any more. To my astonishment, it worked. I asked the coach how it could be that you can hold your breath longer when swallowing water and remember him replying, 'No idea, but it works.' I realized later in my JB practice that the action of swallowing opens the 'throat', a pranic release takes place and the need to breathe reduces.

Refrain

Pranayama is not respiration, but the expansion of Prana. Pranayama is a process not in the physical body but in the pranic body. Prana is not air or breath, but life that enters each embryo and settles in the navel centre; death occurs when Prana, life, leaves.

Pranayama, the expansion of Prana, is a threefold process: (1) the expanding of Prana from its origin in the navel centre outwards; (2) the reversing of Prana back to the navel centre; and (3) the containing of Prana in the navel centre. The threefold process is called vayu, and it happens in the rhythm of the breath, but it is not breath, and it moves in the opposite direction to respiration. Vayu does not move through air tubes but through nadis. The nadis are full of impurities, and pranayama is the purification process. Once the nadis are purified, the vayu stops moving and breath ceases. Prana then remains for prolonged periods in the navel centre where it creates heat, which awakens a dormant pranic force sitting in the base chakra, kundalini. Kundalini rises in the innermost, spiritual nadi, sushumna; when it reaches the top, sahasrara, an enlightened state occurs.

The bandhas are mechanisms for breaking through the granthis situated in sushumna in order to clear the path for kundalini. When kundalini has reached sahasrara, the crown, then samadhi occurs.

Chapter 6

SAMADHI

The purpose of pranayama, as we have seen, is not an increase in lung capacity; it was not practised with respiratory health in mind. Pranayama was practised and taught to purify the pranic body for the awakening of kundalini. The subsequent rising of kundalini, with the help of the bandhas, can eventually reach the crown, sahasrara, which transforms the practitioner into the mysterious state referred to with many different names:

> Rajayoga, Samadhi, Unmani, Manonmani, Amaratva, Laya, Tattwa, Sunya, Asunmya, Parama Pada, Amanasaka, Asdvaita, Niralambha, Niranjana, Jiivanamukti, Sahaja and Turya are all synonyms. (HYP 4, 3-4)

The purpose of pranayama is reaching this state.

All these words indicate a state of fulfilment and bliss, ecstasy, stillness of mind, insight and a connection to the mystery of Being and the universe. These terms generally refer to a temporary state, a state where the practitioner is exclusively absorbed into inner experiences and the mind is eradicated. One is temporarily incapable of engaging in the chores of life, a state defined by absence of outer perception, thought and Ego. Skill and much practice are needed to reach this state.

There is another state described as the goal of Yoga which is named Kaivalya, Moksha, Nirvana, Yoga.

This is a long-term state, if not even the final state – a state defined by detachment, rather than skill. In that state, the practitioner has eradicated the Ego and experiences crystal-clear awareness and compassion.

When the warrior Arjuna asks his teacher Krishna what the signs of final liberations are, he receives the answer:

> Being settled in the Self and being the same in pain or pleasure, (is the enlightened), to whom a clod, a stone or a piece of gold are the same… to whom honour and dishonour are the same, impartial towards friend or enemy… (Bhagavad Gita 14, 24–25)

Ultimate inner freedom is reached, without attachment to anyone and anything. The mental capacity nevertheless functions, and one is perfectly able to continue with ordinary life chores, as the Buddhist proverb says: 'Before kaivalya chop wood and carry water, after kaivalya chop wood and carry water.'

Many English words have been used to describe both states: enlightenment, ecstasy, final freedom, liberation, sainthood… Our modern culture is not familiar with those states; it denies their possibility and therefore does not distinguish between the temporary and final state. The best English translations, in my view, are 'ecstasy' for the temporary samadhi state and 'final freedom' for the lasting kaivalya state. Those two states are certainly related; learning the control that enables samadhi is a prerequisite to eventually reaching the detachment-free kaivalya.

The Patanjali Yoga Sutras name two approaches which, when applied in the practice, will lead to the enlightened states: abhyasa (control of the mind) and vairagya (detachment) (Patanjali 1, 2). Abhyasa is a disciplined training that can lead to samadhi even if one is still attached. In kaivalya, the total Ego-free state has been reached, all attachments are overcome and vairagya is completed, but daily life continues, and the mind is functioning.

The Patanjali Yoga Sutras, the main source of Raja Yoga, describe and instruct samadhi in the first three chapters in detail. The fourth chapter is dedicated to kaivalya, the final step. Once samadhi is experienced, the journey goes on to kaivalya. The Hatha compositions focus on samadhi. Hatha is more a tradition of discipline than detachment. Hatha does not replace samadhi with kaivalya, but sees samadhi as the first step. The second, the ascent to kaivalya, is followed when turning to the Raja practice.

> Hatha Yoga is like a staircase that leads the aspirant to the height of Raja Yoga. (HYP 1, 1)

Both of the most influential Hatha compositions, the HYP and the GS, end their treatise with a chapter on samadhi.

The first part of HYP chapter 4, the chapter on samadhi, revisits the teaching of chapters 1–3 by referring to the practice of asana, pranayama, the kumbhakas and mudras as methods to awaken kundalini, initiating Prana to move in sushumna, which leads to samadhi, the state of the many names (HYP 4, 10–12). Pranayama and all other Yoga practices have no other goal than samadhi.

Further on in the fourth chapter of the HYP, we find more references to Raja Yoga: Hatha and Raja are working hand in hand to reach samadhi. When they become more familiar with the process of reaching samadhi, the practitioner needs to turn fully to the Raja tradition for the final step to kaivalya.

At the end of chapter 4, 66–101, a Hatha-specific method is introduced – a shortcut to the samadhi state, nada. Focus and listening to the inner sound will break through the granthis and purify sushumna and thus stop the senses and mind. The Yogi is absorbed and becomes untouchable, and even death cannot harm them.

The chapter, and thus the whole treatise, ends with the statement:

> As long as marut (synonym of vayu) is not entering the middle (sushumna)…true knowledge can't be gained. (HYP 4, 1134)

Pranayama is the technique to bring the vayu into sushumna and to reach samadhi. Pranayama is one stepping stone towards this mysterious state with many names. From there, Raja Yoga needs to complete the journey to the ultimate and final kaivalya.

CONCLUSION

Pranayama has been lost in translation because our culture is not open to the realization of any processes beyond the anatomical body. Pranayama has turned into a therapy, an approach that is not known in the ancient texts. Therapy is all we want from it; our purely anatomical reality has to function. Our culture as a whole does not formulate the necessity for human development and evolution. The only growth we talk about is economic growth, not spiritual growth. Purifying our subtle existence, reaching a state like samadhi or kaivalya, is meaningless in our culture. Speaking about enlightenment in a Yoga class is almost indecent. We believe that we are our bodies, nothing else, and when those bodies stop functioning, then we are no more. The belief and experience that we still exist when the body ceases to function, has been, and is, upheld by all cultures in all times, with the exception of modern Western culture. That does not mean that everyone living in the West denies an after-life – many people don't – but the culture as a whole has no space for an assumption of a non-physical, ongoing existence. The possibility of having a non-physical consciousness which is not negated by death is not researched or taught, has no space in any curriculum, is not contemplated, is nearly a taboo.

Children are often asked, 'What do you want to do when you are grown up?' No one ever asks, 'Where will you go and what will happen when you die?' Why is that? It should be the most important question as it is inevitably applicable to every living being.

If we were open to the possibility of an ongoing consciousness, then we would have to admit that the way we live our lives might have an effect on our after-life, and that is a no-go area for a culture that has lost any moral base, decency and ethical norms.

I always dedicate some time in my teacher training courses to a discussion on reincarnation, as it is taught in the Bhagavad Gita. Once a student expressed the view that reincarnation is a faith for weak and scared people who do not have the courage to face the finality of death. The other participants managed to convince the student that it is actually the other way round. It is fear that prevents the consideration of a further existence, as a further existence might turn out to be not favourable for those who have lived an Ego-centred life.

This fear is the origin of the insistent denial of any non-physical elements within humanity. When assuming that death is the extinction of the entire living being, then the way a life is lived is irrelevant, and practices that lead to a purified and enlightened state are meaningless. It is more comfortable to deny the possibility and necessity of inner evolution, as this releases us from the responsibility of our actions. It is much more comfortable to reduce a practice like pranayama to a therapy instead of seeing it as it was originally taught, a practice that purifies, completes the practitioner, removes the veil over the inner light and leads to an enlightened state and thus to a blissful life and after-life.

To teach pranayama the original way is not only giving us more benefits and increased effectiveness; it makes us more considerate and open to realities beyond our physical body and limited intellect.

I firmly believe that we Yoga practitioners and teachers need to move beyond saying, 'We don't need the old scriptures, we know better, we have our anatomy.' We need to embrace the sacred teachings, practise them and gain insight from them. From the practice of the sacred teachings, we can learn that life has a purpose, and realize that growing personally, not economically, makes us more alive, happy, kind, mature and connected within this life and for whatever will follow.

Oh Yogi, therefore study, understand and practise the true pranayama.

Glossary

The Sanskrit names of postures are not included; those are not essential for the understanding of Yoga, whereas the following concepts are.

Abhyasa: (practice) a term used in the Yoga Sutras of Patanjali to describe the practice of mental focus.

Adhana: (gate) there are 16 adhanas connected with the 16 petals of vishuddhi; when closed through the practice of jalandhara, bandha attentions cannot escape.

Agni: (fire) one of the five elements, also referring to the inner fire sitting in the middle of the abdomen.

Agni sari: (the invigorator of the inner fire) the practice of drawing the abdominal wall rapidly inwards with empty lungs.

Ajna-chakra: (the wheel of wisdom) the sixth chakra in the middle of the head, often referred to as the third eye.

Akasha: (ether) space, the fifth element.

Anahata-chakra: (the unstuck wheel) the fourth chakra in the middle of the chest, also referred to as the heart centre.

Ananda: (bliss) a state reached when, through Yoga practice, the outer layers are cleared.

Anandamaya kosha: (the sheath of bliss) the most subtle of the human layers, koshas.

Annamaya kosha: (the sheath of food) the physical body.

Antaraya: (impediment) human obstacles preventing the disciplined practice of Yoga, described in the Patanjali Yoga Sutras 1, 30.

Apana: (anus) that field of Prana that pervades the lower abdominal area.

Asana: (seat) Yoga posture, the third of the eight limbs of Yoga as described in the Patanjali Yoga Sutras.

Atman: (the inner Self) the immortal, unchangeable inner consciousness, synonym of Purusha.

Avidya: (ignorance) the first of Patanjali's kleshas (Patanjali 2, 3), the cause for all attachments and duality.

Ayurveda: (ayus = life; veda = knowledge) the Indian science of healing.

Bandha: (bondage) three practices facilitating the rise of Prana in sushumna.

Bastrika: (little bag, bellows) a Hatha Yoga practice stimulating the pranic flow, by contracting the abdominal wall sharply with an exhalation and expanding it strongly during inhalation, like the bellows of a blacksmith.

Bindu: (dot) the point at the upper back of the head where all creational power originates.

Brahma granthi: (the knot of Brahma) the attachment to possessions which is a knot situated in sushumna nadi between the first and the second chakra.

Chakra: (wheel) pranic centres in the body; there are six main ones located on sushumna nadi.

Candra (Chandra): moon.

Citta: (mind) that space where mental activities, vrittis, take place. Defined as having three activities: manas, the ability to register information supplied by the senses; buddhi, the ability to categorize; and ahamkara (I-maker), the creation of the sense of a separate me.

Devangari: the script used from the fourth century CE onwards notating Sanskrit.

Dharana: (concentration) the sixth of Patanjali's eight limbs; focus on one object.

Dhyana: (meditation) the seventh of Patanjali's eight limbs, a prolonged focus on one object.

Dosha: (fault) there are three different doshas, or body types (vata, pitta, kapha), used in Ayurveda for diagnosis and healing.

Drishti: (gaze) a concentration technique where the gaze remains on one point.

Dukha: (the dark space) a term referring to all human suffering.

Granthi: (blockage, knot) a Hatha term for blockages in sushumna caused by attachments.

Guna: (virtue) three basic tendencies (rajas, tamas, sattva), which interact and create the appearance of the universe.

Guru: (the weighty one) a master, teacher.

Ida-nadi: (the Prana conductor called ida) one of the three major energy channels, situated on the left of the central axis.

Jala: (water) one of the five elements; this word is often used in conjunction with neti (nasal washing with water).

Jalandhara bandha: one of the three bandhas, which raises Prana in sushumna from the throat upwards.

Kaivalya: (aloneness) refers to the state when the Self/Purusha is freed from all mind stuff and is in peace and awareness of itself. It is different from samadhi; kaivalya can be maintained in daily life.

Kanda: (bulb, piece) the point of origin of all nadis, which is situated in the middle of the abdomen, experienced as egg-shaped and white.

Kaplabhati: (cleansing the head) a movement of the abdominal wall in the rhythm of the breath, with the aim to clear the sinuses.

Kapha: (phlegm) the body type (dosha) describing a slow, heavy and grounded person.

Karma: (action) any action in life that is in itself neutral but leaves deposits when done in attachment.

Kechari mudra: a mudra that facilitates opening of the pranic body and the rise of kundalini; turn the tip of the tongue up to the roof of the mouth, bring it back to the soft palate and point it up towards ajna chakra.

Kevala kumbhaka: (absolute cessation) the state when breathing stops after an exhalation; the duration can be up to several hours in an accomplished master.

Klesha: (trouble, affliction) referred to in Patanjali 2, 1–10. Obstacles which are the causes of losing the Yoga path. They are forms of attachments, except the first, which is ignorance, the cause of attachments.

Kosha: (sheath) a concept first mentioned in the Taittiriya Upanishad, describing the five layers of human physicality.

Kriya: (synonym of karma, action) kriya-yoga is a term used by different traditions, having quite different meanings; it just means: 'do Yoga by being active'.

Kumbhaka: (pot like) referring to the pause after the exhalation, which can extend with mind control to kevala kumbhaka.

Kundalini: (serpent) the dormant pranic force residing at the mouth of sushumna, which can be awakened through yogic practices.

Laya: (dissolution) absorption; classified by the HYP as a synonym of samadhi.

Mala (two short a's): (impurity) a synonym of klesha; this term is used in the HYP to describe the impurities in the nadis.

Mala (two long a's): (beads, rosary) used for prayer and meditation, having 108 beads.

Manas: (lower mind) that ability in the human to register what the senses perceive.

Manipura chakra: (wheel of the city of jewels) the third chakra, situated in the middle of the abdomen.

Manomaya kosha: (the sheath made of mind) the third layer of human physicality.

Mantra: (manas = mind; tra = save) a sound or combination of sounds used to influence human nature. Some mantras are words with a meaning, others only sounds used for their vibration.

Maya: (magic, illusion) the Indian experience that the universe as perceived by the mind is not the ultimate reality.

Moksha: (liberation) the dissolution of all mental aspects; a synonym of kaivalya.

Mudra: (seal, gestures) Yoga practices that purify nadis to increase the pranic movement.

Muladhara chakra: (the wheel of the root container) the lowest of the energetic centres, sitting in the pelvic floor region.

Nabhi: (navel) the middle of the abdomen, where different pranic events are rooted. It is the location for manipura chakra and also for kanda.

Nada: (sound) different from mantra, as this is not a sound to be chanted, but an existing sound to be listened to in the inner body.

Nadi: (Prana conductor) the pathways in which the pranic life force moves.

Niyama: (observances) the five practices of the second limb of Patanjali's Yoga practices.

Om: the most sacred mantra, expressing the Divinity.

Pingala-nadi: (the brown Prana conductor) one of the three major energy channels, situated slightly right of the central axis.

Pitta: (brass) the body type (dosha) describing a creative, fiery and stable person.

Prajna: (wisdom, insight) a synonym of jnana.

Pralaya: (decay) dissolution, end of the universe.

Prana: (life) the experience of being alive.

prana: the term prana, when transliterated with a lowercase 'p', also refers to the vayu moving in the chest region.

Pranamaya kosha: (the sheath of Prana) the pranic body.

Pranayama: (expansion of prana) the fourth of Patanjali's limbs.

Pratyahara: (withdrawal) the fifth limb of Yoga described in the Yoga Sutras of Patanjali, the control of the senses.

Puraka: (filling) the movement that fills all the nadis. During puraka, which happens during exhalation, the vayu moves back to kanda.

Purusha: (the transcendental Self) in most texts used as a synonym of Atman.

Rajas: (dust) to be coloured, affected; one of the three gunas, the three principles the universe is made out of, discussed in the Bhagavad Gita chapters 14–18. Rajas is the moving forward, pushy, striving element.

Recaka: (purging, expelling) one of the three phases of pranayama, the expansion of the vayus outwards, which happens during the inhalation.

Rudra granthi: (the knot of Rudra) Rudra is a deity, who became assimilated into the god Shiva; rudra granthi is the energetic knot in sushumna, situated between the fifth and sixth chakra. It is formed out of attachment to siddhis.

Sadhu: (virtuous) a saintly person.

Sahasrara: (thousand) the energetic opening at the top of the head, often referred as the seventh chakra. The destination for rising kundalini.

Sahita kumbhaka: (the incomplete kumbhaka) retention, a pause between exhalation and inhalation occurring by the practice of pranayama. As long as an inhalation is still to follow, the kumbhaka is incomplete, and thus sahita.

Samadhi: (enstasy) absorption, the eighth limb in Patanjali Yoga Sutras, the state where the mind is fully controlled.

Samana: (equal, alike) the current of pranic force moving from kanda sideways into the abdominal area and back.

Samnyasa, samnyasin: renunciation, renouncer.

Samskara: (impression) imprints in the mind, learned thought patterns, which create shade over the Self even if the mind is not active. The dissolution of samskaras is one of the last steps to final liberation.

Sattwa: (essence) illumination; one of the three gunas, the state that the Bhagavad Gita describes as the attachment-free state when rajas and tamas are overcome.

Shakti: (power, energy) often used as a synonym of Prana. In the Indian understanding, the universe is created by the merging of consciousness/Shiva and energy/Shakti. That is symbolized in the Indian mythology by the holy marriage of the god Shiva and the goddess Shakti.

Shambhavi mudra: the gaze towards the point between the eyebrows, a mudra that activates ajna chakra.

Shanthi: (peace) can denote any state from mental equilibrium to highest absorption in the Absolute.

Shatkarma: (six acts) used in the Hatha tradition to describe cleansing practices preliminary to pranayama. Those practices are often also named kriyas.

Shruti: (what is heard) revelation; the term is used for verses that were formulated in a state of revelation and gained a sacred status.

Siddha, siddhis: (person with special powers, special powers) an accomplished person and accomplishments; through dedicated Yoga practice, accomplishments can be gained from perfection of body, breath and mind control. Those skills (e.g. levitation, mind reading) are described in chapter 3 in Patanjali.

Smitri: (memory) a term used for epics, traditional verses describing events in Indian history and divine actions. Smriti is distinct from shruti.

Srishti: (creation) the creation of the universe.

Sthiti: (firm) the sustenance of the universe, the process of evolution and maintenance.

Sukha: (joy, ease, the open space) one of the two descriptive words Patanjali uses in 2, 46 to describe how asana need to be performed.

Surya: sun.

Sushumna: (the most gracious) the middle of the three most important nadis, which opens when the breath ceases; kundalini power can then rise up that channel to reach the goal of Hatha Yoga.

Sutra: (thread) a verse; very compact instructions, easy to memorize for a practitioner to practise.

Svadhyaya: (gaining for oneself) the fourth niyama, second of the eight Patanjali limbs of Yoga, instructing the chanting of verses of wisdom.

Svatsistana chakra: (the wheel of one's own abode) the second energetic wheel, situated in the middle of the pelvis.

Tadagi mudra: (the gesture of a water well) a Hatha Yoga practice that frees the vayu flow from impurities by slow contractions of the abdominal wall with the exhalation, like digging a hole in the belly.

Tamas: (darkness) one of the three gunas, refers to the attitude of lethargy, laziness, non-caring.

Tantra: (loom) a Yoga tradition formed in early medieval times studying the pranic body in detail. Tantra became known for its sexual practices.

Tapas: (heat, glow) the discipline and determination needed to be applied to the yogic practice. It is listed in the Patanjali eight limbs as the third niyama.

Udana: (joy) one of the five vayus, the pranic field moving into head, arms and legs and back again.

Ujjayi: (ut = upwards; jayi=conquer) the practice of restricting the throat during breathing to produce a sonorous sound.

Vata: (air) the body type (dosha) describing a light, unstable air person.

Vayu: (wind) the move of pranic fields from kanda through the whole nadi system and back. There are five different frequencies: prana – moving in the chest; apana – moving in the pelvis; samana – moving in the abdomen; udana – moving in head, arms and legs; and vyana – a reserve force potentially active all over the pranic system.

Vedanta: (the Vedas' end) the Yoga school interpreting the teachings of the Vedas, one of the six dharshanas.

Vidya: (knowledge) the seeing of the impermanent core of what there is, that what is missing in the state of avidya (ignorance), which is the cause of all attachments.

Vijnanamaya kosha: (vi = down, into; jnana = wisdom) the sheath made out of wisdom; the fourth of the koshas, the inborn knowing of what the Self and the universe is made out of.

Vishnu granthi: (the knot of Vishnu) the attachment to people and peer pressure, situated as an energetic block in sushumna between the third and the fourth chakra.

Vishuddhi chakra: (vi = down, into; Shuddhi = purification) the fifth energy wheel, situated in the throat.

Vyana: (one of the five vayus) a frequency of prana that moves throughout the whole nadi system.

Yama: (restraint) there are five restraints in the Patanjali eight limbs: ahimsa (non-violence), satya (truthfulness), asteya (non-stealing), brahmacharya (chastity) and aparigraha (non-greed).

Yoga: (union) coming together of two elements.

Bibliography

Burley, Mickel (2000) Hatha Yoga: Its Context, Theory and Practice. Delhi: Motilal Banarsidass Publishers.
Coulter, David (2001) Anatomy of Hatha Yoga. Honesdale, PA: Body and Breath.
Dalrymple, William (2013) Nine Lives: In Search of the Sacred in Modern India. London: Bloomsbury.
Dalrymple, William (1999) The Age of Kali. London: Flamingo.
Desikachar, T.K.V. (1995) The Heart of Yoga: Developing a Personal Practice. Rochester, VT: Inner Traditions.
Desikachar, T.K.V., and Desikachar, Kausthub (2013) Yoga Travali. Chennai: Krishnamacharya Yoga Mandiram.
Easwaran, Eknath (1988) The Upanishads. Arkana.
Feuerstein, Georg (2014) The Bhagavad Gita. Boulder, CO: Shambhala.
Feuerstein, Georg (2001) The Yoga Tradition. Prescott, AZ: Hohm Press.
Feuerstein, Georg (1990) Encyclopedic Dictionary of Yoga. London: Unwin Paperbacks.
Feuerstein, Georg (1989) The Yoga-Sutras of Patanjali, Rochester, VT: Inner Traditions.
Gopalacharlu, S.E. (1894) An Introduction to the Mantra Shastra. Chennai: Theosophical Publishing House.
Gopi, Krishna (1993) Living with Kundalini. Boulder, CO: Shambhala.
Grimes, John (1996) A Concise Dictionary of Indian Philosophy: Sanskrit Terms Defined in English. New York: SUNY Press.
Hewitt, James (1991) The Complete Yoga Book: The Yoga of Breathing, Posture and Meditation. London: Rider.
Hirschi, Gertrud (2000) Yoga in Your Hands. Boston, MA: Weiser Books.
Iyengar, B.K.S. (2005) Light on Life. Emmaus, PA: Rodale.
Iyengar, B.K.S. (1991) Light on Yoga. London: Thorsons.
Jessup, Warwick, and Jessup, Elena (2021) Stories from the Mahabharata: A Sanskrit Coursebook for Intermediate Level. Delhi: Motilal Banarsidass Publishers.
Jessup, Warwick, and Jessup, Elena (2020) Sanskrit: An Introductory Course. Delhi: Motilal Banarsidass Publishers.
van Lommel, Pim (2010) Consciousness Beyond Life: The Science of the Near-Death Experience. New York: HarperCollins.
Van Lysebeth, André (1982) Yoga: für Menschen von Heute. Munich: Mosaik Verlag.
Van Lysebeth, André (1972) Pranayama: The Yoga of Breathing. London: Unwin Paperbacks.

Nair, Anita (2007) The Puffin Book of Magical Indian Myths. New Delhi: Puffin Books India.
Olivelle, Patrick (1996) Upanishads. Oxford and New York: Oxford University Press.
Sinh, Pancham and Vasu, Rai Bahadur Shrisha Chandra (2014) The Forceful Yoga; Being the Translation of Hathayoga-Pradipika, Gheranda-Samita and Shjiva-Samita. Delhi: Motilal Banarsidass Publishers.
Ram, Tulsi [Trans] (2013) Atharvaveda, Volume I. London: UK.
Sabatini, Sanda (2000) Breath: the Essence of Yoga. London: Thorsons.
Sanskrit IGCSE (2019-2024) Literature Set Texts Extracts.
Scaravelli, Vanda (1991) Awakening the Spine. New York: HarperCollins.
Smith, D. John (2009) The Mahabharata. London: Penguin Classics.
Sri Swami Satchidananda (1988) The Living Gita. Yogaville, VA: Integral Yoga Publications.
Sris Chandra Vasu (1976) The Gheranda Samitha. London: Theosophical Publishing House.
Swami Gambhirananda (2013) Eight Upanishads. Kolkata: Trio Process.
Swami Mukthibodananda (1998) The Hatha Yoga Pradipka. India: Bihar.
Swami Mukthibodhananda (1984) Swara Yoga. India: Bihar.
Swami Narasimhananda [Trans] (2024) Yogataravali Sutras. https://devanpillaitoronto.wordpress.com/2024/03/13/yoga-taravali
Swami Niranjanananda Saraswati (2002) Prana Pranayama Prana Vidya. India: Bihar.
Swami Nishchalanandha Saraswati (2003) Ashram Chants. Mandala Yoga Ashram.
Swami Satyadharma (2003) Yoga Chudamani Upanishad. India: Bihar.
Swami Satyananda Saraswati (1998a) Moola Bandha: The Master Key. Yoga Publications Trust.
Swami Satyananda Saraswati (1998b) Yoga Nidra. India: Bihar.
Swami Satyananda Saraswati (1996a) Asana Pranayama Mudra Bandha. India: Bihar.
Swami Satyananda Saraswati (1996b) Kundalini Tantra. India: Bihar.
Swami Satyananda Saraswati (1983) Meditations from the Tantras. India: Bihar.
Swami Svatmarama (1972) Hatha Yoga Pradipika. Madras: Adyar Library and Research Centre.
Swenson, David (1999) Ashtanga Yoga: The Practice Manual. Austin, TX: Ashtanga Yoga Productions.
Vorphal, Frank (2019) Schliemann und das Gold von Troja: Mythos und Wirklichkeit. Berlin: Verlag Galiani.
Wildcroft, Theodora (2020) Post-Lineage Yoga: From Guru to #MeToo. Sheffield: Equinox Publishing.

Articles

Ailani, Ritu (2022) 'Pranayama yoga breathing benefits for health.' Femina, 22 April. www.femina.in/wellness/health/pranayama-yoga-is-the-key-to-perfect-health-224879.html#what-is-pranayama-yoga
Anderson, Sandra (2017) 'Hatha yoga and the Natha yogis.' Himalayan Institute, 14 August. https://himalayaninstitute.org/online/hatha-yoga-natha-yogis
Cleveland Clinic (2024) 'Diaphragmatic Breathing.' https://my.clevelandclinic.org/health/articles/9445-diaphragmatic-breathing
Free Man Creator (2024) 'Embryo in the Womb.' https://anthroposophy.eu/Embryo_in_the_womb#part_of_the_journey_-_descent